T0015596

FOOT REFLEXOLOGY & ACUPRESSURE

A Natural Way to Health through
Traditional Chinese Medicine

By Zha Wei

Better Link Press

This book is edited and designed by the Editorial Committee of *Cultural China* series.

Text by Zha Wei
Translation by Wu Yanting
Design by Wang Wei

Copy Editor: Shelly Bryant
Editor: Cao Yue
Editorial Director: Zhang Yicong

Senior Consultants: Sun Yong, Wu Ying, Yang Xinci
Managing Director and Publisher: Wang Youbu

ISBN: 978-1-60220-164-4

Address any comments about *Foot Reflexology & Acupressure: A Natural Way to Health through Traditional Chinese Medicine* to:

Better Link Press
99 Park Ave
New York, NY 10016
USA

or

Shanghai Press and Publishing Development Co., Ltd.
F 7 Donghu Road, Shanghai, China (200031)
Email: comments_betterlinkpress@hotmail.com
Printed in China by Shanghai Donnelley Printing Co., Ltd.

1   3   5   7   9   10   8   6   4   2

The material in this book is provided for informational purposes only and is not intended as medical advice. The information contained in this book should not be used to diagnose or treat any illness, disorder, disease or health problem. Always consult your physician or health care provider before beginning any treatment of any illness, disorder or injury. Use of this book, advice, and information contained in this book is at the sole choice and risk of the reader.

Contents

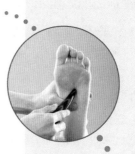

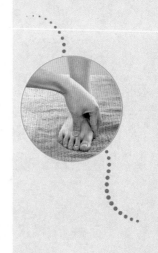

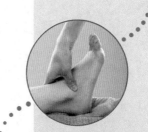

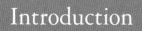

The practices of foot reflexology and acupressure have become well accepted as more people are increasingly aware of the importance of maintaining one's health. In general, foot therapy includes two parts, foot bath and foot reflexology, with the latter being most common. There are 77 reflex zones and 65 acupoints in the feet, each corresponding closely to a human internal organ or tissue. Stimulating these acupoints or the pathological reflex zones will regulate the functions of the *zangfu* organs and alleviate a variety of diseases, which will help people stay healthier.

Many of the reflex zones are located in the feet. Which should I massage? Should I do both? If I am coughing constantly, should I massage when I am coughing, or simply massage on a daily basis? My hands get tired doing reflexology. Is there a way to reduce the stress on my hands? What should I do if I cannot accurately locate the acupoints and reflex zones in my feet? This book will address these questions that have been raised by readers, outlining detailed steps including the duration of each massaging, the number of sessions needed to treat a disease, and how many sessions a course of treatment requires. In addition, the book will teach you how to use a reflexology stick, which not only relieves the stress on the hands, but also generates better therapeutic effects.

The book features pictures of real persons and computer graphics to show the locations of acupoints and reflex zones. They are not only beautiful to look at and easy to find, but are also highly accurate. The book has included foot reflexology and acupressure for 53 common diseases, alongside ten additional types of therapeutic approaches. You will learn to administer foot reflexology and acupressure simply by following the picture, with one image dedicated to each step. Massaging at home for a few minutes every morning and evening, for yourself or for your family, will bring both physical and mental relaxation to those who suffer from exhaustion.

Your health journey begins with a single step.

Chapter One

Understanding Foot
Reflexology and Acupressure

In the streets and lanes of many cities, there are foot massage parlors of varying sizes. Foot massage (also referred to as foot reflexology and acupressure) is becoming a lifestyle. Why don't we bring foot reflexology home from the parlor, doing it at home to take control of your own health? Learning to do foot reflexology and acupressure will help enhance your ability to care for your health and wellbeing. You will not only be able to promptly relieve pain for yourself, but also for your loved ones, which will in turn strengthen the bond among family members and add to it the small pleasures of life, even as your overall health and wellbeing are improved.

1. Benefits

Doing foot reflexology and acupressure regularly can promote the flow of vital qi and the circulation of blood, regulate the functions of the internal organs, and remove blockages in the meridian paths. This will help eliminate disease and pathogens, remove blood stasis, facilitate blood flow, and build up the body's vital energy.

Promoting Blood Circulation, Removing Blood Stasis and Toxins

Foot reflexology and acupressure can improve the blood circulation of various parts of the feet and the related reflex zones. The stimulation causes the blood vessels to dilate, the blood flow to accelerate, and more blood to pass through these passages. Foot reflexology primarily serves to improve the blood circulation of the reflex zones of the excretory organs such as the kidneys, ureter tube, and bladder, which in turn improves the functions of corresponding organs. In addition, foot reflexology invigorates the functions of the lungs and bronchi, inducing an increased exchange of oxygen and carbon dioxide in the lungs and bronchi. This is how foot reflexology and acupressure work to detox, promote blood circulation, and dissipate blood stagnation.

Restoring the Balance of Yin and Yang

Traditional Chinese medicine teaches that a disease develops mainly because of the imbalance of yin and yang in the body. By stimulating acupoints or reflex zones, certain biological signals are generated and transmitted through the meridian system or the nervous system to the corresponding *zangfu* organs, tissues, and other organs, thus triggering a process that restores the balance between yin and yang and alleviate a host of diseases. Foot reflexology and acupressure are effective in regulating the functions of related organs in two ways, instead of just one. For example, stimulating the Zusanli acupoint can treat both constipation and diarrhea.

Regulating the Functions of the *Zangfu* Organs

The internal organs of the human body have corresponding points found in the feet. Six of the 12 meridians originate from the feet, where the *Zusanyin* meridians (the foot yin meridians) start and the *Zusanyang* meridians (the foot yang meridians) end. More than 60 acupoints spread across both feet and connect the internal and external environments. By stimulating the reflex zones or acupoints of the feet, foot reflexology and acupressure regulate the functions of the *zangfu* organs, thereby preventing the occurrence of diseases and alleviating a variety of illnesses.

Generating Endogenous Drug-Like Factors

Foot reflexology and acupressure can induce biochemical and biophysical changes in the human body. These changes are called "endogenous drug-like factors," substances produced by the organism itself in response to signals that call for treatment. They do no harm to the human body and play a role no exogenous medication can replace, and therefore result in unexpected therapeutic effects. They play a particularly prominent role in boosting the human immune system and fighting infection.

2. Tools

Doing foot reflexology and acupressure with the fingers alone is likely to lead to overexertion, and your hands become tired and sore quickly. As a result, the intensity of stimulation will decrease and the result of the reflexology will be affected. For this reason, it is advisable that you use a reflexology stick.

Using tools, such as a reflexology stick, a buffalo horn, or even a wooden stick, will double the results with half the effort. A reflexology stick made of buffalo horn is comfortable to the

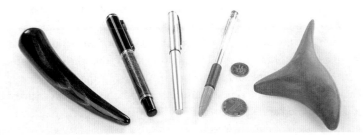

Fig.1 Tools for foot reflexology and acupressure.

touch and easy to carry around. In addition, it has the properties of cooling the blood, detoxifying the body, promoting the circulation of blood, relieving muscle and joints stress, and boosting cellular immunity. It has a distinctive effect on neurasthenia and effectively relieves muscle pain.

3. Duration and Number of Treatments

When doing foot reflexology and acupressure, it is crucial that you massage for the right amount of time. The duration of each stimulation should be determined based on factors such as the type of disease, its severity and the patient's particular constitution.

Generally, the massaging of each acupoint or reflex zone lasts 2 to 3 minutes, or 30 to 50 stimulations. However, for reflex zones such as the kidneys, ureter, bladder, lungs and bronchi, you must massage each for 5 minutes, or 100 to 200 stimulations, to ensure that the excretory function be strengthened so that toxic substances can be removed smoothly from the body.

Reflexology for a patient with severe heart disease should last no more than one minute on the heart reflex zone. In total, no more than ten minutes is needed when taking into account the massaging of other reflex zones and acupoints. For patients with severe diabetes and kidney disease, the total massage time should not exceed 10 minutes. The massage of each reflex zone on the spine should be about 2 to 3 minutes.

It is recommended that you do a massage once or twice daily. To achieve better results, you should do it once every day over a long period of time. If you massage once every day, it is better to do it at a fixed time. If you massage twice daily, it should be done once in the morning and once at night before bed. Do not massage after a full meal or on an empty stomach. Each session should last 30 minutes. For an ordinary disease or condition, 10 sessions make up one course of treatment. Having recovered from the disease after performing foot reflexology and acupressure, you should continue the massage for some time to ensure that the improvements achieved are maintained and so that your physical fitness will be strengthened and the risk of recurrence reduced.

4. Basic Techniques

When performing reflexology on yourself, you should adopt a sitting posture, on a bed, the floor, a couch, or a chair, according to your preference. Rest your left foot on your right knee, with the sole facing upward, and massage with your right hand. Massage the right foot after you are done with the left.

Foot reflexology and acupressure require that the intensity and number of stimulations grow incrementally and the duration of a stimulation also increases gradually. It is advised that each session lasts about 30 minutes. The following is a list of eleven commonly-used techniques.

Pressing with Thumb Pad

Place the pad (friction ridge side) of the thumb on a specific acupoint or pathological reflex zone of the foot and press down gradually, with the pressure increasing from light to heavy. The pressure should grow incrementally in a firm and persistent manner.

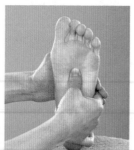

Kneading

Place the pad of the thumb on a specific location. With the elbow as an anchor point, move the forearm deliberately so the mobility of the wrist will allow the fingers to move in a soft and gentle motion. This technique is often used in coordination with pressing.

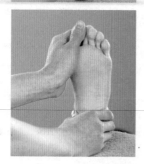

Pressing with Thumb Tip

Place the tip of the thumb or the knuckle of the thumb on acupoint or pathological reflex zone of the foot and hold it down forcefully, gradually going from light to heavy.

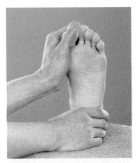

Pushing

Place the tip or pad of the thumb on a specific area of the foot and apply pressure by moving in a single direction in a straight line. The tip or pad of the thumb remains in contact with the skin surface for the duration of the move, which should be done slowly but evenly.

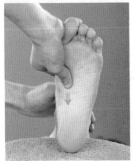

Circular Rubbing

Rubbing in a circular motion is done by the index, middle, and ring fingers. Lay these fingers on a specific area of the foot and use the mobility of the wrist as the center to administer pressure through the metacarpals and phalanges as they move rhythmically in a circular motion. The rubbing should remain slow, gentle, and coordinated.

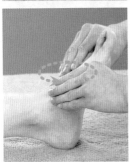

Grasping

By pressing against one another, the thumb and the index and middle fingers, or the thumb and the four remaining fingers, pinch and lift a certain area or acupoint of the foot in rhythmic movements. The application of force should be gentle, moving from light to heavy, and the motion should be mild and consistent.

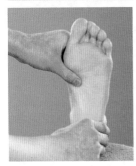

Traction

One hand holds up the patient's heel while the other hand grips the phalange of the patient's big toe and pull it gently first, gradually increasing the force until you feel a loosening sensation at the ankle. For nervous patients, a little swing of the foot before traction will help them relax.

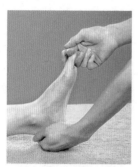

Percussing

Percussing refers to the stimulation method of hitting or beating the acupoint on the foot like raindrops. It can be applied on all acupoints in the foot, especially in the areas that are not sensitive. When percussing is performed, exertion of force should be abrupt and brief and any dragging or whipping should be avoided.

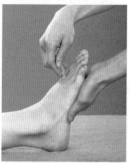

Rubbing To and Fro

This method of stimulation requires that the minor thenar be placed on the larger reflex zones. Apply a proper amount of lubricating oil to both protect the skin and strengthen the therapeutic effect.

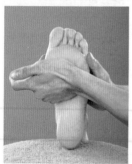

Nipping

Among the techniques associated with foot reflexology, nipping exerts the strongest stimulation. With all the force concentrated in the tip of the thumb, the nail side of the thumb stabs or presses an acupoint. The local area is then gently kneaded to relieve the pain generated by the action. Nipping is often used for acute or severe problems. Be careful to avoid damaging the skin.

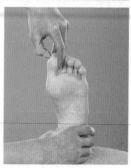

Rotating

One hand holds the heel of the patient while the other hand grips the big toe to make rotating movements in the ankle joint. The direction and amplitude of rotation should not go beyond the physiological limits of the patient.

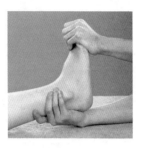

5. Treatment Sequence

It is important to follow certain sequences when doing foot reflexology in order to avoid compromising the effect of the treatment. In general, foot reflexology should be done in the following sequence:

(1) Before each foot reflexology session, check the patient's heart condition. If the patient suffers from severe heart disease, decrease the intensity and the duration of stimulation. Make sure that you check the patient's heart condition again at the beginning of each course of foot reflexology treatment to determine the intensity of the treatment and note the condition of the disease.

(2) After deciding which acupoints to work with, perform the treatment on both feet, the left foot first, followed by the right.

(3) Massage reflex zones of the body organs such as the kidneys, bladder, ureter, lungs, and bronchi to enhance the functions of the urinary and respiratory systems so metabolic wastes can be effectively removed from the body.

(4) Massage the selected reflex zones and acupoints in turn. If time permits, massage both feet thoroughly, following this sequence: the sole, the medial and lateral sides, the dorsum, and the lower leg. Press each point or zone three times.

(5) Finally, massage once again the reflex zones for the kidneys, bladder, ureter, lungs, and bronchi.

This sequence is particularly appropriate for diseases of a more complex nature and chronic diseases that are known to have a long development. However, not all the diseases and conditions follow the same sequence. For instance, for ailments such as sprained joints, locked shoulders, migraines and toothache, massage should be conducted directly on one or a few reflex zones or acupoints that are related to the disease. Details of each alternative will be discussed in Chapters Three and Four.

6. Intensity of Stimulation

Foot reflexology is a comprehensive therapy that involves the treatment of various disorders by applying pressure to acupoints and the reflex zones of the feet that pertain to particular parts of the body. Through foot reflexology, pain caused by a variety of diseases can be alleviated and the development of diseases can be averted so that the body will stay in good working order. For most of the acupoints and reflex zones, the general rule is, the stronger the pressure, the more severe the pain and the better the results. In other words, no result will be achieved if no pain is felt. This is particularly true in the case of pain related to bones, joints, muscles, and ligaments. Greater pressure must be applied in order to achieve the desired results. However, excessive pressure should be avoided, as it can harm the periosteum. In addition, the application of pressure should increase incrementally, from light to heavy, until it reaches the limit of the patient's tolerance.

A small number of people are especially sensitive to pain and have a very low tolerance of pain. When doing foot reflexology for this type of patients, observe their facial expressions. If the patient turns pales, it is a sign that the limit has been reached, and you should stop applying pressure immediately or take a break. Let the patient rest for a moment before resuming the massage when the patient is ready.

7. Cautions

(1) Foot reflexology should be conducted in a quiet, sheltered place without the disturbance of wind or strong light. Never practice foot reflexology in the open. Keep the room well-ventilated, clean and tidy.

(2) Keep practicing foot reflexology as a routine so as to acquire the endurance you need, the skills with hand movements, and proficiency in the various techniques. Keep your hands clean and warm, and trim your nails regularly.

(3) Before each foot reflexology session, let the patient take a short rest and be informed of the things he or she needs to know. It is advised that the individual takes a foot bath for 15 to 30 minutes in tolerably warm water that covers ankles. He or she should then lie supine on the bed and let the whole body relax.

(4) When doing foot reflexology for a patient, the reflexologist should assume a sitting position with a towel on the knee and rest

the patient's foot on the reflexologist's knee. An examination of the patient's feet should be conducted to find the painful points in the reflex zone. Use the tip of a ballpoint pen or a stick to test it. When the individual feels a sharp twinge, then you have found the right point.

(5) Do not do foot reflexology after overeating, on a full stomach, or within an hour after taking a bath or after overexertion.

(6) After foot reflexology, drink no less than 250 to 500 ml of warm water. For patients with severe heart conditions and kidney problems, drink no more than 150 ml water. Seniors and children should also drink less than the recommended volume.

(7) Avoid massaging protruding parts of the bones and places where there is little subcutaneous tissue, so the periosteum does not get hurt.

(8) After foot reflexology, do not wash the feet in cold water. Remove the massage oil on the feet with tissue paper and put on a pair of socks to keep warm. Before going to bed, wash the feet clean of massage oil and take a foot bath in warm water, making sure that you soak your feet in the warm water for 15 minutes (fig. 2).

(9) When certain reactions occur during a foot reflexology treatment, the patient should inform the reflexologist inmediately so the reflexologist can deal with it promptly, or opt for an alternative method of massaging, if necessary.

(10) Those who attempt self-massage should progress gradually in due order and strictly follow the operational requirements.

(11) For severe illnesses, professional medical treatment is paramount, and foot reflexology and acupressure should only be used as auxiliary therapies.

(12) Effective foot reflexology and acupressure therapies call for the individual's resilience and perseverance.

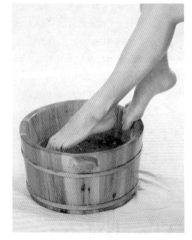

Fig.2 Soak your feet in the warm water befor going to bed.

8. Normal Reactions

In addition to certain expected therapeutic effects following the treatment, foot reflexology and acupressure will also trigger other reactions. The following is a list of normal reactions.

(1) Increased sleep. During the course of foot reflexology therapy, some people feel great fatigue and often grow very sleepy. Sleep at night tends to be deeper and dreams become more frequent. Such reactions indicate that the patient's physiological functions are adjusting to a state of "protective repression."

(2) Increased perspiration. Sweat may give off unpleasant smell, or feet that are not sweaty may suddenly become sweaty after foot reflexology. Perspiration is conducive to the excretion of body toxins and metabolic wastes. Increased sweating in the feet is indicative of the improved blood circulation in the feet, of boosting the sensitivity of the acupoints to the stimulations by foot reflexology, and the effect of health maintenance.

(3) Frequent urination. In the course of foot reflexology, the receiver tends to generate more urine, which often gives off odourous smell. If the urine is left to stand for some time, sediments will appear, which is a sign of the excretion of body toxins and deposits.

(4) Frequent bowel movements. After a foot reflexology treatment, the patient will have frequent bowel movements, and the volume of stools will increase. The stools give off a stronger odor and the patient may notice increase flatulence, which may even occur as the foot reflexology is being conducted. All this is indicative of increased intestinal movements that are helpful to clearing and alleviating disorders caused by the obstruction of the flow of qi in the internal organs.

(5) Increase in secretions of the mucus membrane in the nose, eyes, and respiratory tracts.

(6) For female patients, the appearance of leukorrhea, increased discharge of leukorrhea, or leukorrhea giving off a stronger unpleasant smell.

(7) Increased thirst or water intake.

These reactions are all within the normal range, indicating that the patient is restoring the metabolical functions and the waste is being excreted from the body.

9. Unusual Reactions

Foot reflexology exerts strong stimulation to the corresponding organs and tissues, which can trigger unusual reactions in some patients. Common reactions may include:

(1) After foot reflexology and acupressure treatment, a patient with severe kidney disorders could start to excrete urine that is black or red in color. This happens because the body's energy is clearing the yang stagnation caused by cold and damp and dividing nutrients and waste material so that the body toxins and wastes are excreted. If the foot reflexology continues, this symptom will disappear and everything will return to normal.

(2) Some patients with back pain will feel even greater pain after the foot reflexology, but the pain will subside significantly a day later. This is a reaction to the massage that facilitates the blood circulation and clears the channels and collaterals.

(3) For some people with varicose veins, their veins will appear even thicker, which is in fact a good sign, because the stagnation in the blood is removed and the blood flow is smooth, the effect of removing the old and bringing in the new. At this point, keep doing the foot reflexology.

(4) After foot reflexology, some individuals will experience swollen ankles, especially for those who have lymphatic stasis. Do not worry. Keep doing the foot reflexology, and the swelling will subside when the flow of body fluids is normal.

If unusual reactions to the foot reflexology persists, the patient should see a doctor.

10. Indications

All therapies have their limits. This is also true of foot reflexology and acupressure. Based on analyses of years of clinical experience and thousands of case studies, we have found that foot reflexology and acupressure are applicable primarily to the following conditions and disorders:

(1) Evident results for neurosis, including hypothalamic vegetative nerve system dysfunction, dysfunctions of a variety of internal organs, and a host of neuropathic pains. This is because foot reflexology therapy regulates the equilibrium of excitation

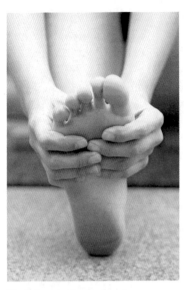

Fig.3 Foot reflexology and acupressure play a critical role in regulating the physiological functions of the human body.

and depression in the central nervous system and has an evident effect on blocking the sense of pain.

(2) Evident effect in the treatment of chronic gastrointestinal diseases. Foot reflexology and acupressure boost the functions of digestion and absorption of the digestive system.

(3) Evident results for all sorts of allergic diseases, such as allergic asthma, allergic rhinitis, and allergic dermatitis. Foot reflexology has a great effect on restoring the balance of neuroendocrine system and greatly improving the adrenocortical function to induce a function similar to corticosteroids (e.g. cortisone and prednisone).

(4) Evident effect on a variety of infections, such as mastitis, lymphadenitis, lymphangitis, upper respiratory inflammation, and asthmatic bronchitis. These are indications that foot reflexology and acupressure boost the functions of the body's immune system.

(5) Effective in treating venous vasculitis of the lower extremities and stasis dermatitis, evident that foot reflexology and acupressure effectively improve the blood circulation.

Briefly, foot reflexology and acupressure play a critical role in regulating the physiological functions of the human body and work effectively with a variety of functional diseases. They also have a certain effect on some organic diseases, but they should not be used alone, but as a major auxiliary to professional medical treatment.

11. Contraindications

Foot reflexology and acupressure have a wide range of indications. They work well with a variety of diseases and incur no side effects.

However, as with all therapies, foot reflexology and acupressure have their limits, beyond which such practices produce no effect. Caution should be exercised when dealing with certain disorders and diseases. The following is a list of contraindications.

(1) Some surgical conditions, such as acute peritonitis, perforation of intestine, acute appendicitis, bone fracture, joint dislocation, etc.

(2) A variety of acute infectious diseases, such as typhoid fever, cholera, epidemic meningitis, epidemic encephalitis B, hepatitis, tuberculosis, syphilis, gonorrhea, and AIDS.

(3) Acute toxicity, such as food poisoning, carbon monoxide poisoning, drug poisoning, alcohol poisoning, snakebite, and rabies.

(4) Acute diseases with high fever, such as septicaemia.

(5) A variety of hemorrhage, such as brain hemorrhage, stomach bleeding, uterus bleeding, and other visceral bleeding.

(6) Diseases such as acute myocardial infarction, severe renal failure, and heart failure.

(7) For a woman during her menstruation period and pregnancy.

(8) During the active phase of an individual's mental illness.

The disorders and diseases are often characterized as urgent conditions, since changes can happen in the blink of an eye and therefore should be treated in a timely manner. Any delay might adversely affect the chances of recovery. Those in critical conditions are usually physically weak and fragile and cannot withstand the pain of a massage. In addition, foot reflexology facilitates blood circulation, which may result in serious consequences for some patients.

To people with these contraindications, it is advised that they go for professional medical treatments through medication and surgery. When their conditions are stable or alleviated, foot reflexology and acupressure can be used as an auxiliary means of therapy to reinforce the treatment and shorten the duration of the illness.

Chapter Two

Acupoints and Reflex Zones in the Foot

The human body is an organic whole, and all the component parts are closely related. When a disorder occurs to one organ or tissue, then, another organ or tissue may also be affected. For example, when an individual is affected by liver qi stagnation, he or she will experience symptoms known as dysfunction of the spleen in transportation, including loss of appetite, semiliquid stools, or abdominal distention. All of these symptoms are the result of transverse invasion of the hyperactive liver's qi and the invasion of the spleen meridian. When treating the disease of one organ, therefore, it is important that the patient not only identify the cause of the disease, but that he or she also understand how it affects other organs and tissues. Only with such a holistic perspective can one determine what acupoints and reflex zones to stimulate in order to treat the root causes.

1. Meridians and Acupoints

As the basis of TCM theory, the meridian system can actually be observed in real life, though no research has yet uncovered any convincing evidence of its physical form. To put it simply, the meridian system is like a traffic network spreading across the human body, consisting of channels designed exclusively to supply qi (vital energy) and blood to every part of the body. Among them, the principal channels are called *jing* (meridians), and the branching vessels connecting the principal channels and connected with one another are called *luo* (collateral). Serving the five visceral organs (*wuzang*) and six bowel organs (*liufu*), they crisscross the human body, connecting the surface and the internal organs, as well as the top and the bottom, in an organic whole. Through the circulation of qi and blood, they provide nutrition to sustain the organic livelihood of the human body.

There are fourteen meridians in the human body. They are:
- Taiyin Lung Meridian of the Hand (LU)
- Yangming Large Intestine Meridian of the Hand (LI)
- Yangming Stomach Meridian of the Foot (ST)
- Taiyin Spleen Meridian of the Foot (SP)
- Shaoyin Heart Meridian of the Hand (HT)
- Taiyang Small Intestine Meridian of the Hand (SI)
- Taiyang Bladder Meridian of the Foot (BL)

- Shaoyin Kidney Meridian of the Foot (KI)
- Jueyin Pericardium Meridian of the Hand (PC)
- Shaoyang Sanjiao Meridian of the Hand (TE)
- Shaoyang Gallbladder Meridian of the Foot (GB)
- Jueyin Liver Meridian of the Foot (LR)
- Conception Vessel (CV)
- Governing Vessel (GV)

The foot is traversed by a large number of meridians. Meridians affecting such organs as the stomach, gallbladder, bladder, liver, spleen and kidneys all go through the feet and have some points connected to each organ there.

Body Length Measurement

1. Use Thumb Length	2. Use Middle-Finger Length	3. Use Four Fingers Closed Together
The width of the patient's thumb joint is 1 cun. This is applicable for locating the acupoint on four limbs with vertical cun.	With the patient's middle sections of the bent middle finger as measurement, the distance between two inner crease tips is taken as 1 cun, which is mostly applicable for locating acupoints on four limbs with vertical cun and on the back with horizontal cun.	With the index finger, middle finger, ring finger, and small finger stretched straight and closed, measure at the level of the large knuckle (the second joint) of the middle finger. The width of the four fingers is 3 cun.

1cun

1cun

3cun

Located along the pathways of the meridians and collaterals, acupoints are usually places where nerve endings concentrate or locations where thicker nerve fibers travel. When you feel discomfort or pain, it is the acupoints that send out the pain signals. The acupoints situated along the pathways of the fourteen principal meridians are called "meridian points." In addition, there are acupoints in certain fixed location that have special effects for treatment. Those are called "extra-ordinary points." These acupoints are not isolated on the surface of your skin, but are closely connected to organs and tissues deep inside your body. Therefore, in a sense, acupoints reflect problems inside your body, and they are working points for treating those problems. You can locate these acupoints with body length measurement (see the table on facing page).

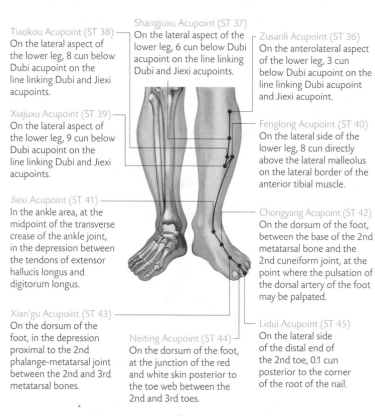

Tiaokou Acupoint (ST 38)
On the lateral aspect of the lower leg, 8 cun below Dubi acupoint on the line linking Dubi and Jiexi acupoints.

Xiajuxu Acupoint (ST 39)
On the lateral aspect of the lower leg, 9 cun below Dubi acupoint on the line linking Dubi and Jiexi acupoints.

Jiexi Acupoint (ST 41)
In the ankle area, at the midpoint of the transverse crease of the ankle joint, in the depression between the tendons of extensor hallucis longus and digitorum longus.

Xian'gu Acupoint (ST 43)
On the dorsum of the foot, in the depression proximal to the 2nd phalange-metatarsal joint between the 2nd and 3rd metatarsal bones.

Shangjuxu Acupoint (ST 37)
On the lateral aspect of the lower leg, 6 cun below Dubi acupoint on the line linking Dubi and Jiexi acupoints.

Neiting Acupoint (ST 44)
On the dorsum of the foot, at the junction of the red and white skin posterior to the toe web between the 2nd and 3rd toes.

Zusanli Acupoint (ST 36)
On the anterolateral aspect of the lower leg, 3 cun below Dubi acupoint on the line linking Dubi acupoint and Jiexi acupoint.

Fenglong Acupoint (ST 40)
On the lateral side of the lower leg, 8 cun directly above the lateral malleolus on the lateral border of the anterior tibial muscle.

Chongyang Acupoint (ST 42)
On the dorsum of the foot, between the base of the 2nd metatarsal bone and the 2nd cuneiform joint, at the point where the pulsation of the dorsal artery of the foot may be palpated.

Lidui Acupoint (ST 45)
On the lateral side of the distal end of the 2nd toe, 0.1 cun posterior to the corner of the root of the nail.

Fig.4 Yangming Stomach Meridian of the Foot (ST).

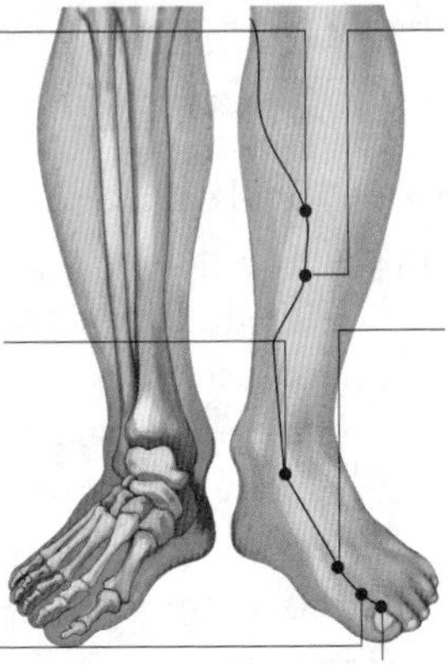

Zhongdu Acupoint (LR 6)
On the medial aspect of
the lower leg, 7 cun directly
above the medial malleolus,
in the middle of the medial
side of the tibia.

Ligou Acupoint (LR 5)
On the medial aspect
of the lower leg, 5 cun
directly above the medial
malleolus, in the middle of
the medial side of the tibia.

Zhongfeng Acupoint (LR 4)
On the ankle, anterior to
the medial malleolus, in the
depression on the medial
border of the tendon of
tibialis anterior.

Taichong Acupoint (LR 3)
On the dorsum of the foot,
in the depression anterior to
the articulation of the bases
of the 1st and 2nd metatarsal
bones, or at the point where
the pulsation of the dorsal
artery of the foot may be felt.

Xingjian Acupoint (LR 2)
On the dorsum of the foot, at the
junction of the red and white skin
posterior to the margin of the web
between the 1st and 2nd toe.

Dadun Acupoint (LR 1)
On the toe, on the lateral side of the
distal phalange of the big toe, about 0.1
cun posterior to the corner of the nail.

Fig.5 Jueyin Liver Meridian of the Foot (LR).

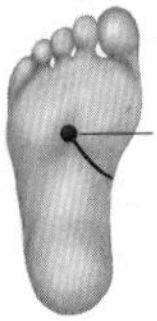

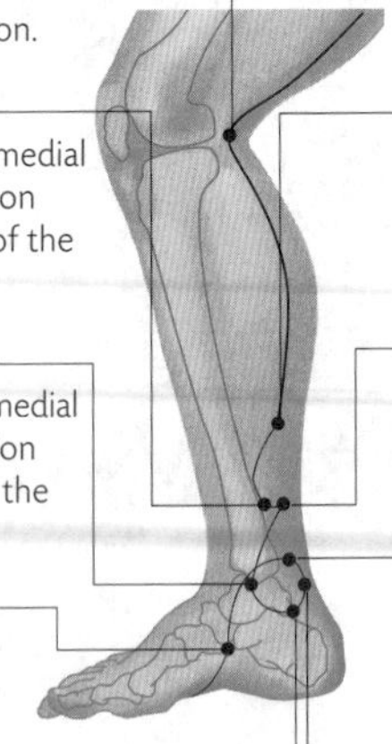

Yongquan Acupoint (KI 1)
In the depression formed
on the sole when the foot
is in plantar flexion.

Yin'gu Acupoint (KI 10)
With the knee flexed, on the
popliteal transverse crease, on
lateral border of the tendons of
the semitendinosus.

Jiaoxin Acupoint (KI 8)
2 cun directly above the medial
malleolus, in the depression
on the posterior border of the
medial side of the tibia.

Zhubin Acupoint (KI 9)
On the medial side of the lower
leg, 5 cun directly above Taixi
acupoint between the soleus
and the tendo calcaneus.

Zhaohai Acupoint (KI 6)
1 cun directly below the medial
malleolus, in the depression
on the inferior border of the
medial malleolus.

Fuliu Acupoint (KI 7)
2 cun directly above the
medial malleolus, anterior
to the Achilles tendon.

Ran'gu Acupoint (KI 2)
Inferior to the tuberosity
of the navicular, at the
junction of the red and
white skin.

Taixi Acupoint (KI 3)
In the depression between
the prominence of the
medial malleolus and the
calcaneal tendon.

Shuiquan Acupoint (KI 5)
1 cun directly below Taixi acupoint,
in the depression on the medial
border of the calcaneus.

Dazhong Acupoint (KI 4)
Posterior and inferior to the medial
malleolus, in the depression on the
anterior border of the Achilles tendon.

Fig.6 Shaoyin Kidney Meridian of the Foot (KI).

Yinlingquan Acupoint (SP 9)
On the medial aspect of the lower leg, in the
depression between the inferior margin of
the medial condyle of the tibia and the medial
border of the tibia.

Lou'gu Acupoint (SP 7)
6 cun directly above the
medial malleolus on the
posterior margin of the
medial side of the tibia.

Shangqiu Acupoint (SP 5)
On the ankle, anterior
and inferior to the medial
malleolus, in the depression
which lies at the midpoint
of the line linking the
tuberosity of navicular and
the prominence of the
medial malleolus.

Taibai Acupoint (SP 3)
On the metatarsal bone, in
the depression proximal to
the 1st metatarsophalangeal
joint at the junction of the
red and white skin.

Diji Acupoint (SP 8)
3 cun below Yinlingquan,
on posterior margin of the
medial side of the tibia.

Sanyinjiao Acupoint (SP 6)
3 cun directly above the
medial malleolus on the
posterior margin of the
medial side of the tibia.

Gongsun Acupoint (SP 4)
On the anterior and
inferior border of the base
of the 1st metatarsal bone,
at the junction of the red
and white skin.

Yinbai Acupoint (SP 1)
On the medial side of the
big toe, 0.1 cun posterior
to the corner of the nail.

Dadu Acupoint (SP 2)
On the medial side of the big
toe, in the depression distal to
the 1st metatarsophalangeal
joint, at the junction of the
red and white skin.

Fig.7 Taiyin Spleen Meridian of the Foot (SP).

Qiduan Acupoint (EX-LE 12)
At the midpoints of the
tips of all toes, 0.1 cun from
the free margin of the nail,
altogether 10 acupoints on
the left and right foot.

Duyin Acupoint (EX-LE 11)
On the sole of foot, at
the midpoint of the distal
metatarsal bone and
interphalangeal joint of
the 2nd toe.

Dannang Acupoint (EX-LE 6)
On the lateral side of the lower
leg, 2 cun directly below the
small head of the fibula.

Lanwei Acupoint (EX-LE 7)
On the lateral side of the lower
leg, 5 cun below the depression
lateral to the patellar ligament,
one cun from the anterior side
of the tibia.

Waihuaijian Acupoint (EX-LE 9)
On the ankle, at the prominent
point of the lateral malleolus.

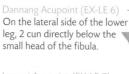
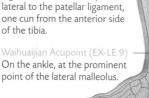

Fig.8 Extraordinary Points.

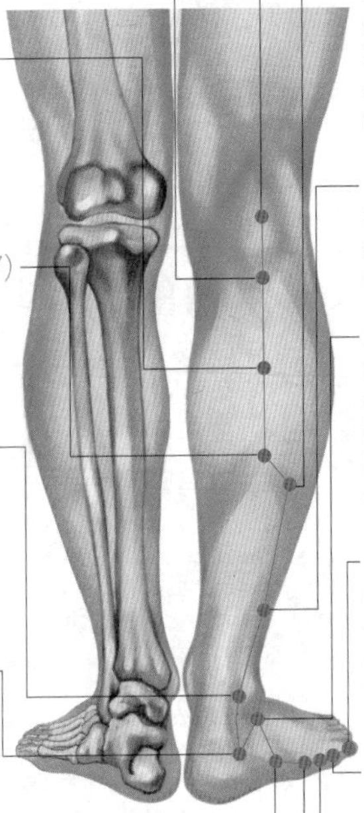

Heyang Acupoint (BL 55)
On the posterior aspect of
the lower leg, 2 cun below
the popliteal transverse crease
between the medial and lateral
head of the gastrocnemius
muscle.

Chengjin Acupoint (BL 56)
5 cun below the popliteal
transverse crease, between
the bellies of the two
gastrocnemius muscles.

Chengshan Acupoint (BL 57)
At the junction of the belly
and tendon of the two
gastrocnemius muscles.

Kunlun Acupoint (BL 60)
Behind the ankle joint, in
the depression between
the prominence of the
lateral malleolus and the
Achilles tendon.

Pucan Acupoint (BL 61)
Directly below Kunlun
acupoint, lateral to the
calcaneus bone at the
junction of the white
and red skin.

Jinmen Acupoint (BL 63)
On the lateral side of the foot, directly below
the anterior border of the lateral malleolus, in
the depression on the inferior border of the
cuboid bone, posterior to the tuberosity of the
5th metatarsal bone.

Jinggu Acupoint (BL 64)
At the junction of the red and white skin
anterior and inferior to the tuberosity of the
5th metatarsal bone.

Weizhong Acupoint (BL 40)
With the knee flexed, at the
midpoint of the popliteal
transverse crease.

Feiyang Acupoint (BL 58)
7 cun directly above Kunlun
acupoint, at the junction
of the lateral and inferior
border of the gastrocnemius
muscle and the Achilles
tendon.

Fuyang Acupoint (BL 59)
3 cun directly above Kunlun
acupoint between the
fibula and Achilles tendon.

Shenmai Acupoint (BL 62)
Directly below the lateral
malleolus, in the depression
between the posterior
border of the lateral
malleolus and the calcaneus.

Zhiyin Acupoint (BL 67)
On the lateral side of the
distal phalange of the
small toe, 0.1 cun posterior
to the corner of the nail.

Zutonggu Acupoint (BL 66)
On the lateral side of
the distal end of the 5th
metatarsophalangeal joint,
at the junction of the red
and white skin.

Shugu Acupoint (BL 65)
At the junction of the
red and white skin
proximal to the 5th
metatarsophalangeal joint.

Fig.9 Taiyang Bladder Meridian of the Foot (BL).

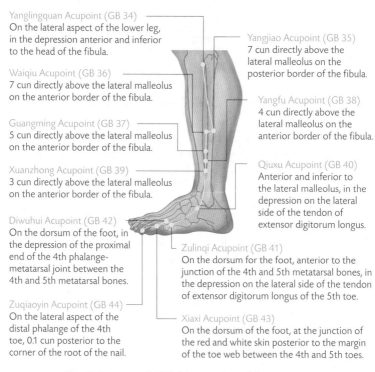

Yanglingquan Acupoint (GB 34)
On the lateral aspect of the lower leg, in the depression anterior and inferior to the head of the fibula.

Waiqiu Acupoint (GB 36)
7 cun directly above the lateral malleolus on the anterior border of the fibula.

Guangming Acupoint (GB 37)
5 cun directly above the lateral malleolus on the anterior border of the fibula.

Xuanzhong Acupoint (GB 39)
3 cun directly above the lateral malleolus on the anterior border of the fibula.

Diwuhui Acupoint (GB 42)
On the dorsum of the foot, in the depression of the proximal end of the 4th phalange-metatarsal joint between the 4th and 5th metatarsal bones.

Zuqiaoyin Acupoint (GB 44)
On the lateral aspect of the distal phalange of the 4th toe, 0.1 cun posterior to the corner of the root of the nail.

Yangjiao Acupoint (GB 35)
7 cun directly above the lateral malleolus on the posterior border of the fibula.

Yangfu Acupoint (GB 38)
4 cun directly above the lateral malleolus on the anterior border of the fibula.

Qiuxu Acupoint (GB 40)
Anterior and inferior to the lateral malleolus, in the depression on the lateral side of the tendon of extensor digitorum longus.

Zulinqi Acupoint (GB 41)
On the dorsum for the foot, anterior to the junction of the 4th and 5th metatarsal bones, in the depression on the lateral side of the tendon of extensor digitorum longus of the 5th toe.

Xiaxi Acupoint (GB 43)
On the dorsum of the foot, at the junction of the red and white skin posterior to the margin of the toe web between the 4th and 5th toes.

Fig.10 Shaoyang Gallbladder Meridian of the Foot (GB).

2. Reflex Zones

There are 77 reflex zones on the feet. By massaging the reflex zones connected to the brain (head), headache symptoms will subside immediately. Massaging the reflex zone connected to human reproductive gland will improve dysmenorrhea and irregular menstruation. If you suffer from stomachaches, abdominal distention, and indigestion, try the reflex zone connected to the stomach, and the symptoms will be alleviated quickly.

Three Major Types of Reflex Zones and Their Functions

In terms of the functions of the reflex zones in the feet, there are three types, basic reflex zones, symptomatic reflex zones, and auxiliary reflex zones.

Basic Reflex Zones: Mainly including those connected to organs such as the kidneys, urinary tract, bladder, lungs and bronchi. They are the most important reflex zones and have to be massaged at the beginning and the end of each foot reflexology session. The purpose of this massage is to strengthen the body's excretion functions in order to eliminate toxins and metabolic wastes from the body.

Symptomatic Reflex Zones: The areas that directly relate to the symptoms exhibited by the patient. In a patient with rhinitis, for example, this is the nose zone, while in a patient with an upper respiratory tract infection, it is the zone of the lung and bronchus, and in a patient with benign prostatic hyperplasia, it is the prostate zone. For patients with gallbladder infections, the symptomatic reflex zones are the gallbladder and liver zones.

Auxiliary Reflex Zones: Also called Pertaining Reflex Zones, as they could be the pathological areas where the patient's disorders originate. The treatment will be most effective if these reflex zones are accurately located and treated.

Reflex Zone Selection for Treatment

In selecting reflex zones, it should be noted that a rich knowledge of traditional Chinese medicine, Western medicine, and clinical experience are used together. The following is a list of five commonly utilized methods for selecting reflex zones. For the convenience of non-professional readers, this book has listed all the acupoints and reflex zones pertaining to each symptom.

Selection based on traditional Chinese medical theory: Utilizing theories of the yin-yang and the five elements, the relations of the *zangfu* organs and the internal and external circumstances to determine reflex zones and acupoints to work on. It is advised that the best practice is to select only a few, at most three.

Selection via the pathological nature of an ailment: Infectious diseases, cancer, and some chronic diseases are all related to disorders in the immune system that needs to be strengthened. Therefore, reflex zones such as the lymph glands, the spleen, the tonsils, and the groin should be selected for treatment in order to boost the immune system.

Selection by hand-foot correlation: Due to the lack of representation of peripheral areas from the knees to the toes and the elbows to the fingers, the selection of treatment points in those areas follows the correlations of the hands and feet. For example, to treat pain in the knee, the reflex zones to the elbow joint and the upper arm will be selected and massaged.

Selection based on symptoms: These reflex zones are selected based on where the ailments originate. For example, the symptomatic reflex zone of a toothache is the reflex zones to the upper and lower jaws. Auxiliary reflex zones are also chosen for attention. In this case, the brainstem is the auxiliary reflex zone because its reticular formation performs the sensory perception and motor activity communicating pain. Another auxiliary reflex zone is that of the brain. Through massage, the brain will secrete more endorphins, thus effectively alleviating the pain.

Selection based on anatomical relations: Reflex zones are selected because they are closely associated with the symptomatic reflex zones. For example, in addition to the cerebrum and cerebellum, headaches are also associated with other reflex zones, such as the frontal sinuses, trigeminal nerve, and the cervical spine. Diseases of the stomach can be worked with reflex zones for organs such as the stomach, the esophagus and the duodenum.

Locations of Reflex Zones

Brain (head): On the pads of the distal phalanges of big toes. The left side of the brain is reflected in the right foot, while the right side of the brain is on the left foot.

Frontal sinus: On the soles of both feet, within 1 cm range from the tips of the five toes. The reflex zone to the left frontal sinus is on the right foot, while that of the right frontal sinus is on the left foot.

Cerebellum and brainstem: On the plantar side of big toes, lateral to the base of the proximal phalange. The left side of the cerebellum and the brainstem is reflected on the right foot, while the right side of the cerebellum and the brainstem is on the left foot.

Pituitary gland: At the midpoint (leaning to the medial side) of the pad of the big toes (in the depth of the reflex zone to the brain).

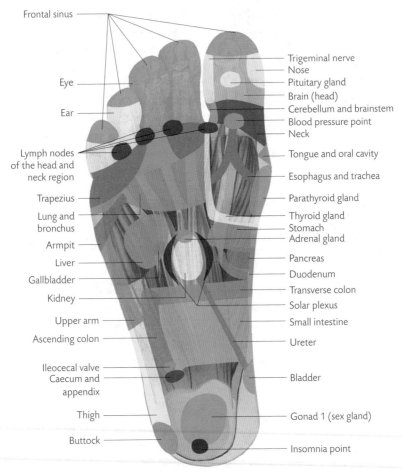

Fig.11 Reflex zones on the plantar side (or the sole) of the right foot.

Trigeminal nerve: On the lateral side of the distal phalange of the big toe, anterior to the reflex zone of the cerebellum and brainstem. The reflex zone of the left trigeminal nerve is on the right foot, while that of the right trigeminal nerve is on the left foot.

Neck: At the plantar side of the base of the big toe. The reflex zone of the left side of the neck is on the right foot, while that of the right side of the neck is on the left foot.

Eye: On both feet, at the phalange and the base of the 2nd and 3rd toes (including both the plantar and dorsal side). The left eye is

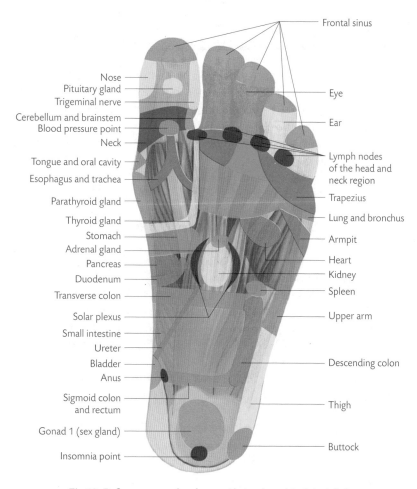

Fig.12 Reflex zones on the plantar side (or the sole) of the left foot.

reflected on the right foot, while the right eye is on the left foot.

Ear: On both feet, at the middle and base of the 4th and 5th toes (including both the plantar and dorsal side). The left ear is reflected on the right foot, while the right ear is on the left foot.

Trapezius: On the soles of both feet, the transverse area about 1 cun-wide inferior to the reflex zones of the eye and ear.

Thyroid gland: On the soles of both feet, the band between the 1st and 2nd metatarsal bones, and the connecting band on the 1st metatarsal.

Parathyroid gland: On the soles of both feet, in the depression anterior to the phalange-metatarsal joint of the 1st toe.

Lung and bronchus: Posterior to the trapezius, in the strip about one cun wide from the thyroid gland reflex zone extending to the shoulder reflex zone. The bronchi sensitive area is situated in the area starting in the middle of the lung and bronchus reflex zones and extending to the 3rd phalange.

Stomach: In the region posterior to the 1st phalange-metatarsal joint, about one cun wide.

Duodenum: On the soles of both feet, in the proximal end of the 1st metatarsal bone, inferior to the reflex zone to the stomach.

Pancreas: On the soles of both feet, in the lower-middle section of the 1st metatarsal bone at the junction of the reflex zones of the stomach and duodenum.

Liver: On the sole of the right foot, inferior to the reflex zone of the lung and bronchus between the 4th and 5th metatarsal bones, as well as the corresponding regions of the dorsal side of the foot.

Gallbladder: On the sole of the right foot, draw a vertical line between the 3rd and 4th toes and then a horizontal line on the reflex zone to the shoulder. The reflex zone to the gallbladder is where the two lines cross.

Solar plexus: On the soles of both feet, in the region among the 2nd, 3rd and 4th metatarsal bones and around the kidney and the stomach reflex zones.

Adrenal gland: On the soles of both feet, between the 2nd and 3rd metatarsal bones, in the depression posterior to the phalange-metatarsal joints and near the reflex zone to the kidney.

Kidney: On the soles of both feet, 1/2 to the proximal end of the 2nd and 3rd metatarsal bones, in the depression anterior to the center of the sole.

Ureter: On the soles of both feet, in a 1-cun-long arc shaped area from the reflex zone to the kidney to the reflex zone to the bladder.

Bladder: Anterior and inferior to the medial malleolus, inferior to the medial aspect of the navicular bone on both feet, next to the abductor of the big toe.

Small intestine: On the soles of both feet, in the depression situated between the cuneiform and calcaneus bones, surrounded by the reflex zones to the ascending colon, transverse colon, descending colon, sigmoid colon, and rectum.

Caecum and appendix: On the sole of the right foot, on the anterior border of the calcaneus bone, close to the lateral side.

Ileocecal valve: On the sole of the right foot, on the anterior border of the calcaneus, close to the lateral side, posterior to the reflex zone to the caecum.

Ascending colon: On the sole of the right foot, lateral to the reflex zone of the small intestine, parallel to the lateral border of the foot, on the strip from the anterior border of the calcaneus to the base of the 5th metatarsal bone.

Transverse colon: On the soles of both feet, the transversing strip at the junction of the bases of the 1st to 5th metatarsal bones, the 1st to 3rd cuneiform bones (i.e., the medial, intermediate and lateral cuneiform bones) and the cuboid bone, across the soles of the feet.

Descending colon: On the sole of the left foot, the vertical strip parallel to the lateral side of the foot from the 5th metatarsal base on the lateral border of the cuboid bone to the lateral and anterior side of the calcaneus bone.

Sigmoid colon and rectum: The strip on the left sole, anterior to the calcaneus bone.

Anus: On sole of the left foot, the medial side of the rectum reflex zone on the anterior border of the calcaneus bone, close to the lateral border of the medial abductor hallucis.

Heart: On the sole of the left foot, inferior to the reflex zone of the lung and bronchus and between the 4th and 5th metatarsal bones, parallel to the reflex zone to the shoulder.

Spleen: On the sole of the left foot, one cun inferior to the reflex zone of the heart, between the 4th and 5th metatarsal bones.

Gonad 1 (sex gland): On the soles of both feet, in the middle of the calcaneus.

Buttock: On the soles of both feet, on the lateral area of the calcaneal tuberosity, in connection with the reflex zone to the thigh.

Thigh: On the soles of both feet, at the strip from the reflex zone to the buttock to the junction of the cuboid bone and the 5th metatarsal bone.

Upper arm: On the lateral border of the both soles of the feet, the strip lateral to the 5th metatarsal bone.

Blood pressure point: On both feet, in the middle of the reflex zone to the neck.

Esophagus and trachea: On the soles of both feet, superior and inferior to the metatarsophalangeal joint of the big toe, next to the reflex zone to the stomach above.

Armpit: On the soles of both feet, the underside of the reflex to the shoulder on the dorsal side of the foot, the strip shaping like a banana, from the lateral border stretching diagonally to the distal end of the space between the 4th and 5th metatarsal bones.

Lymph nodes of the head and neck region: On the soles and dorsa of both feet, in the fossa of the base of each phalange.

Tongue and oral cavity: On the soles of both feet, on the medial border of the base of the distal phalange of the big toe, inferior to the phalangeal joints of the big toe, adjacent to the medial side of the blood pressure point.

Insomnia point: On the soles of both feet, in the middle of the calcaneus bone, posterior to the reflex zone to gonad 1 (sex gland).

Nose: On the medial side of the pad of the big toe, extending to the root of the nail, anterior to the first phalangeal joint. The reflex zone to the left side of the nose is on the right foot and that of the right side of the nose on the left foot.

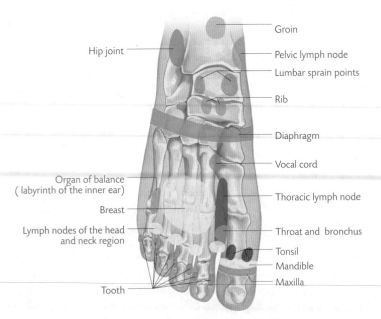

Fig.13 Reflex zones of the dorsal side of the foot.

Thoracic lymph node: On the dorsa of both feet, between the 1st and 2nd metatarsal bones.

Organ of balance (labyrinth of the inner ear): In the distal end 1/2 of the space between the 4th and 5th metatarsal bones.

Breast: On the dorsa of both feet, in the quadrilateral area shaped by the 2nd, 3rd and 4th metatarsal bones.

Diaphragm: On both feet, the strip sweeping across the dorsal side of the metatarsal bones, cuneiform joint and metatarsal bones, and cuboid bone.

Tonsil: On the dorsa of both feet, on the 2nd phalange of the big toe on both sides of the tendon.

Mandible: The strip inferior to the transverse crease on the dorsal side of the inter-phalangeal joint of the big toe.

Maxilla: The strip superior to the transverse crease on the dorsal side of the phalange joints of the big toe.

Throat and bronchus: In the depression posterior to the dorsal side of the junction of the 1st and 2nd metatarsophalangeal joints.

Groin: On the dorsa of both feet, about one cun superior to the reflex zone to the pelvic lymph nodes.

Shoulder blade: On the dorsa of the feet, the proximal 1/2 of the 4th and 5th metatarsal bones, reaching out to the cuboid bone to form the shape of a fork.

Rib: On the dorsa of both feet, the reflex zone to the medial aspect of the rib cage is situated in the area between the 1st cuneiform bone and the navicular bone, and that of the lateral aspect of the rib cage is in the area between the 3rd cuneiform bone and the cuboid bone.

Lumber sprain points: On the dorsa of the feet, in the depressions on both sides of the junction between the 2nd metatarsal bone and the 2nd cuneiform bone, posterior to the reflex zone to the rib.

Tooth: On both sides of each phalangeal joint of the feet.

Vocal cord: On the dorsa of both feet, in the depression anterior and inferior to the junction of the bases of the 1st and 2nd metatarsal bones, between the 1st and 2nd metatarsal bones.

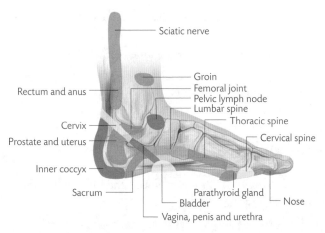

Fig.14 Reflex zones on the medial (or inner) aspect of the foot.

Femoral joint: In the curved area below both medial malleoli.

Pelvic lymph node: Anterior to both medial malleoli, in the depression between the talus and the navicular bone.

Prostate and uterus: In the triangle area posterior and inferior to both medial malleoli.

Vagina, penis and urethra: On the medial aspects of both heels, extending diagonally, backwards and upwards, from the reflex zone to the bladder, in the space between the talus and calcaneus.

Cervical spine: At the 2nd phalange, medial side of the big toe on both feet.

Thoracic spine: On the medial arches of both feet, at the metatarsal and cuneiform joint inferior to the 1st metatarsal bone.

Lumbar spine: On the medial arches of both feet, inferior to the 1st cuneiform bone and the navicular bone, adjoining the reflex zone of thoracic vertebra below and the reflex zone of sacrum above.

Sacrum: On the medial arches of both feet, in the stretch from the lower end of the talus to the calcaneus, with the lumbar spine reflex zone before it and the inner coccyx reflex zone behind it.

Inner coccyx: On the medial aspects of both calcanei of the feet, in the stretch extending diagonally along the calcaneus tuberosity backward and upward.

Cervix: Posterior and inferior to the medial malleoli, the extension of the reflex zones for the ureter.

Rectum and anus: In the medial aspect of the lower leg, between the back of the tibia and the tendon, the strip about 3 cun superior to the posterior of the medial malleolus.

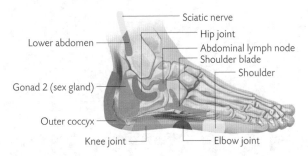

Fig.15 Reflex zones on the lateral (or outer) aspect of the foot.

Knee joint: On the lateral sides of both feet, in the triangle depression of the calcaneus bone between the 5th metatarsal bone and the calcaneus.

Gonad 2 (sex gland): The right triangle area posterior and inferior to the lateral malleolus.

Hip joint: The arches inferior to the lateral malleolus of both feet.

Abdominal lymph node: In the depression between the talus and the navicular bone, anterior to both lateral malleolus.

Outer coccyx: Lateral to the calcanei on both feet, in the strip stretching along the calcaneus tuberosity.

Elbow joint: On the lateral aspects of both feet, the area between the tuberosity of the 5th metatarsal bone and the prominence of the cuneiform bone.

Lower abdomen: On the posterior and lateral side the fibula on both feet, in the strip about 4 thumb-breadths stretching backward from the lateral malleolus.

Shoulder: On the lateral side of the soles of both feet, on the prominence of the 5th phalange and metatarsal joint. The left shoulder reflex zone is on the right foot, while the right shoulder reflex zone is on the left foot.

Sciatic nerve: Levelling the medial and lateral malleoli, the strip extending along the posterior borders of the tibia and fibula and reaching the knee joint.

Chapter Three

For Treatment
of Common Ailments

It is often said, "Your feet are the root of life, and foot reflexology can heal problems throughout the body." Pains and diseases will be alleviated if you simply take a foot bath and massage certain points on your feet before going to bed every day. More importantly, when you do foot reflexology and acupressure at home, there are no side effects to the body, but one usually suffers when taking medicine. Reflexology and acupressure produce immediate results for some acute diseases and pains of various kinds. For some chronic diseases, the results can be good too, as long as you persist in practicing foot reflexology and acupressure for a sustained period of time.

1. Diabetes

Foot reflexology and acupressure have certain healing powers in treating Type 2 diabetes. For instance, they are effective for diabetic patients with high glucose and suger level of 3+ or above in the urine. When foot reflexology treatment is first started, the patient should not stop the medication he or she is taking. As the sugar levels in the blood and urine are lowered, the patient can begin to reduce the amount of medication until it is time to come to a complete stop.

In the course of foot reflexology treatment, attention should be paid to controlling the diet. The patient should rigorously follow the diabetic dietary restrictions, such as taking three meals a day at regular intervals with a fixed amount of food, and taking less sugar-rich food and more protein-rich legumes and vegetables instead. This should be accompanied by regular assessments of the sugar levels in the patient's blood and urine and with regular and appropriate exercise. The patient should also avoid overexertion and fatigue.

Prescription
Do foot reflexology and acupressure to the reflex zones listed below on both feet (except the spleen reflex zone). Start with the left foot, then the right. Stimulate the reflex zones until they feel a distending pain. Do this once daily. For more severe cases, the treatment should be done once in the morning and once in the

evening, with a duration of ten days for a course of the treatment. After three to four courses, when the symptoms have improved, you can reduce the frequency to once daily or once every other day. When the symptoms have disappeared, continue doing the same for a month or two to further advance the improvements achieved.

Steps
1. Press with thumb tip the pituitary gland reflex zone 100 times.
2. Press with thumb tip the reflex zones of the adrenal gland and the kidney 100 times each.
3. From toe to heel, push and press the ureter reflex zone 100 times.

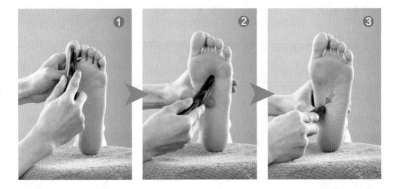

4. Press with thumb tip the bladder reflex zone 100 times.
5. From the medial side to the lateral side of the foot, push and press the reflex zone of the lung and bronchus 100 times each.
6. Press with thumb tip the pancreas reflex zone 200 times.

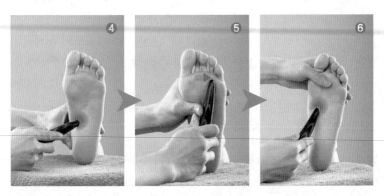

7. Press with thumb tip the reflex zones of the spleen and stomach 100 times each.
8. Press and knead the solar plexus reflex zone for 2 minutes.
9. Starting with the left foot, first from inside to outside and from toe to heel, push and press each of the reflex zones of the transverse colon, descending colon, sigmoid colon, and rectum 60 times each. Then work the right foot from heel to the toes and from outside to inside, push and press the reflex zones of the ascending colon and transverse colon 60 times each.

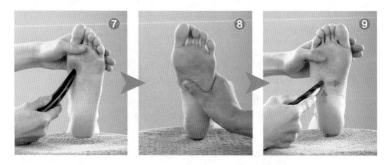

Conclusion: Repeat Steps 2, 3 and 4, but decrease the number of stimulations by half. The treatment should end when this is finished.

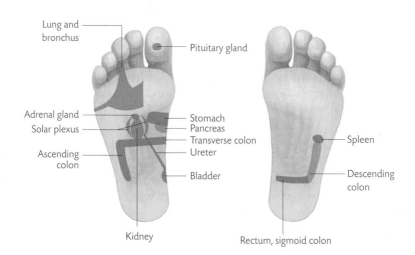

2. Hypertension

Chinese medicine holds that hypertension is mainly a disorder of the liver and kidneys that arises from emotional disturbances, eating disorders, and internal damage and consumptive disease. Therefore, prevention and cure of this disease through foot reflexology and acupressure mainly focuses on regulating and nursing the liver and kidneys, supplemented by balancing yin and yang.

Patients taking anti-hypertensive drugs should not stop medication when they start foot reflexology. As the symptoms have improved, the amount of medication can be reduced accordingly, following doctor's advice, but regular checks of blood pressure should be continued. Hypertensive patients should make sure that they have adequate sleep while undergoing foot reflexology and acupressure. They should exercise regularly and with appropriate intensity, keep a balance of work and rest, stay on a simple and bland diet with little animal fats and internal organs, and quit smoking and alcohol consumption.

Prescription
Do foot reflexology and acupressure once or twice daily, allowing three months for each course of treatment. If your blood pressure returns to normal after three months, the foot stimulation can be reduced to once daily or once every other day.

Steps
1. Press with thumb tip in turn the reflex zones of the kidney, the liver, the adrenal gland and the bladder 100 times each. It is recommended that the intensity of stimulation should produce a distending pain in the local area.
2. Push and press the ureter reflex zone 100 times from toe to heel at a rate of 30 to 50 times per minute.
3. From the medial side to the lateral side of the foot, push and press the reflex zone of the lung and the bronchus 100 times each, at a rate of 30 to 50 times per minute.
4. Press and knead acupoints such as the Yongquan, Taixi, Zhaohai, Taichong, Zusanli, Fenglong, and Taibai 30 times each, until there is distending pain in the local area.

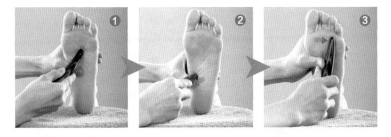

5. Press with thumb tip the reflex zones of the brain (head), the pituitary gland, the neck, the solar plexus, the heart, and the blood pressure point 50 times each, until there's distending pain in the local area.

6. From heel to toe, push and press the thyroid gland reflex zone 50 times, at a rate of 30 to 50 times per minute.

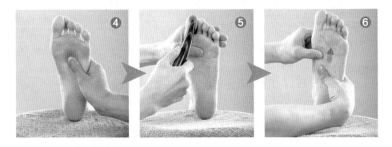

Conclusion: Repeat Steps 1, 2 and 3, reducing the number of stimulations by half. The treatment is concluded when this is finished.

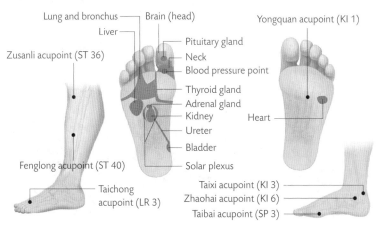

Lung and bronchus —— Brain (head)
Liver ——
Zusanli acupoint (ST 36)
Yongquan acupoint (KI 1)
—— Pituitary gland
—— Neck
—— Blood pressure point
—— Thyroid gland
—— Adrenal gland
—— Kidney   Heart ——
—— Ureter
—— Bladder
Fenglong acupoint (ST 40)
—— Solar plexus
—— Taichong acupoint (LR 3)
Taixi acupoint (KI 3) ——
Zhaohai acupoint (KI 6) ——
Taibai acupoint (SP 3) ——

3. Hypotension

TCM teaches that most chronic diseases are the result of asthenia syndrome. They are caused by the weakening of the transporting functions of the spleen and stomach, deficiencies in the liver and kidney, and insufficient qi and blood, all of which leads to hypotension accompanied by systemic symptoms.

The treatment of hypotension should start with identifying the root cause of the disease and adopting treatment strategies that eradicate the cause. Acute hypotension can not be treated with foot reflexology. Patients with hypotension are advised to lead a regular life, take a diet of more nutritious food, keep a balanced emotional state, quit smoking and drinking alcohol, and do appropriate exercises such as taking walks and practicing tai chi.

Prescription

Doing foot reflexology and acupressure twice daily, allowing three months for a course of treatment. If the patient's blood pressure returns to normal after three months, decrease the frequency of foot reflexology treatment to once daily.

Steps

1. Press with thumb tip in turn the reflex zones of the kidney and bladder 100 times each until a distending pain is felt in the local area.
2. From toe to heel, push-press 100 times the reflex zone of the ureter at a rate of 30 to 50 times per minute, until a distending pain is felt in the local area.
3. From the medial side to the lateral side of the foot, push-press the reflex zone of the lung and bronchus 50 times each, until a

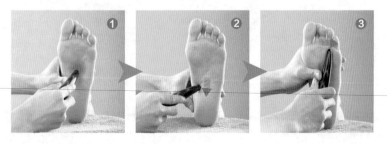

distending pain is felt in the local area.

4. Press with thumb tip the reflex zone to the organ of balance 100 times, and the reflex zones for the brain (head) and adrenal gland 50 times each.

5. From heel to toe, push-press the reflex zone for the thyroid gland 50 times.

6. Press-knead acupoints such as the Taixi, Taichong, Zusanli, and Sanyinjiao 30 times each, and rub the Yongquan acupoint untill the center of the sole generates a warm sensation.

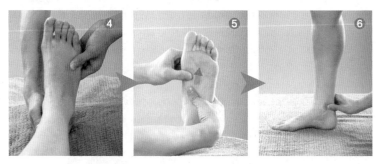

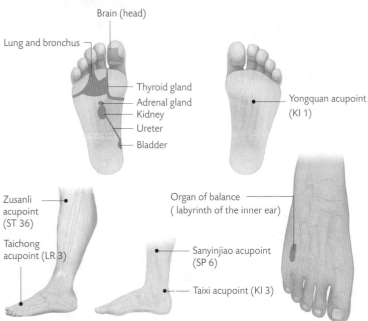

Brain (head)

Lung and bronchus

Thyroid gland
Adrenal gland
Kidney
Ureter
Bladder

Yongquan acupoint (KI 1)

Zusanli acupoint (ST 36)

Taichong acupoint (LR 3)

Organ of balance (labyrinth of the inner ear)

Sanyinjiao acupoint (SP 6)

Taixi acupoint (KI 3)

4. Arteriosclerosis

Stimulating acupoints and zones related to their disease will help regulate the dilation and constriction of the blood vessels and reduce the buildup of cholesterol and triglycerides in a patient's body, preventing the worsening of arteriosclerosis. In the course of the foot reflexology treatment, the patient should consume foods that are low in both cholesterol and animal fat, along with foods that are light but rich in Vitamin C. Patients who also have hypertension should restrict the consumption of salt. Avoid overeating and overdrinking, quit smoking and alcohol, maintain a balanced emotional state, and avoid overexertion. It is recommended that the patient practices tai chi.

Prescription
Do foot reflexology and acupressure once daily. Keep in mind that foot reflexology is only an auxiliary treatment to a major medical treatment of arteriosclerosis.

Steps
1. Press with thumb tip the reflex zones of the kidney, adrenal gland and bladder in turn 100 times at an intensity level that generates a distending local pain.
2. From toe to heel, push-press in turn the reflex zones of the ureter and thyroid gland 100 times each, at a rate of 30 to 50 times per minute.
3. From the medial side to the lateral side of the foot, push-press the reflex zones of the lung and bronchus 100 times each, at a rate of 30 to 50 times per minute.

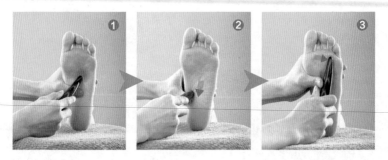

4. Press-knead acupoints such as the Yongquan, Taixi, Sanyinjiao, Taichong, and Zusanli 30 times each, at an intensity level that generates a distending local pain.
5. Press with thumb tip the reflex zones of the brain (head), pituitary gland, parathyriod gland, neck, solar plexus, heart, and cervical spine 50 times each.

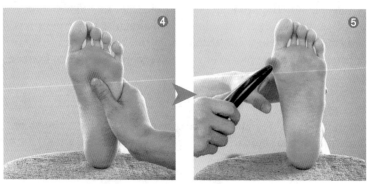

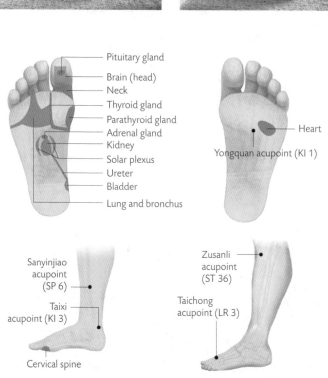

Pituitary gland
Brain (head)
Neck
Thyroid gland
Parathyroid gland
Adrenal gland
Kidney
Solar plexus
Ureter
Bladder
Lung and bronchus

Heart
Yongquan acupoint (KI 1)

Sanyinjiao
acupoint
(SP 6)
Taixi
acupoint (KI 3)
Cervical spine

Zusanli
acupoint
(ST 36)
Taichong
acupoint (LR 3)

5. Headaches

Foot reflexology and acupressure work quite well for headaches caused by hypertension, migraines, vascular headaches, flu-and-cold-related headaches, and other headaches arising from unknown causes.

People suffering from long-term headaches should maintain a simple and bland diet. They should lead a regular life, avoid stress and emotional swings, and abstain from smoking, alcohol, and raw or frozen food. They should engage in appropriate physical exercise, such as jogging or tai chi.

Prescription
Do foot reflexology and acupressure once daily for a course of 3 months. If your headache subsides to almost normal after the three-month treatment, you can reduce the massage to once every other day and continue doing it for one more course to maintain these results.

Steps
1. Press with thumb tip the reflex zones of the kidney, the adrenal gland, and the bladder in turn 100 times each. The intensity level should be sufficient to produce a distending pain in the local area.
2. From toe to heel, push and press the reflex zone of the ureter 100 times at a rate of 30 to 50 times per minute.
3. From the inside edge to the outside edge of the foot, push and press the reflex zone of the lung and bronchus 100 times each, at a rate of 30 to 50 times per minute.

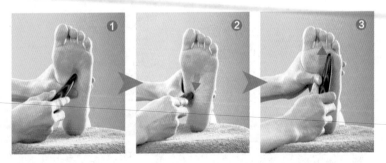

4. Press and knead the Taichong, Taixi, Taibai, Sanyinjiao, and Yongquan 30 times each. The intensity level should be sufficient to produce a distending pain in the local area.
5. Press with thumb tip the reflex zones of the brain (head), the cerebellum, the brainstem, the trigeminal nerve, the lymph nodes of the head and neck region, the solar plexus, the liver, and the pituitary gland, 50 times each. The intensity level should be sufficient to produce a distending pain in the local area.

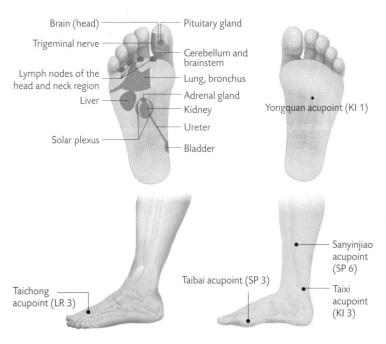

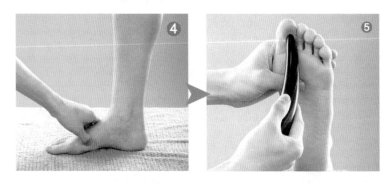

Brain (head)

Trigeminal nerve

Lymph nodes of the head and neck region

Liver

Solar plexus

Pituitary gland

Cerebellum and brainstem

Lung, bronchus

Adrenal gland

Kidney

Ureter

Bladder

Yongquan acupoint (KI 1)

Taichong acupoint (LR 3)

Taibai acupoint (SP 3)

Sanyinjiao acupoint (SP 6)

Taixi acupoint (KI 3)

6. Vertigo

Patients must cooperate with doctors to identify the cause of the vertigo and remain actively engaged in treating the primary disease. Foot reflexology and acupressure are supplementary to treatments by medical professionals. Clinical treatment shows that inner ear vertigo, labyrinthitis, motion sickness, vertigo caused by insufficient blood supply to the basilar artery, and vertigo due to systemic diseases can be treated quite effectively with foot reflexology and acupressure, in combination with traditional Chinese medicine.

Prescription
Do foot reflexology and acupressure once daily for a month for a full course of treatment. The overall treatment can last three to four courses.

Steps
1. Rub the Yongquan acupoint until the center of the sole generates a sense of warmth. The patient, while doing the massage, should breathe naturally and not hold the breath. Administer force evenly. Massage at a rate of 80 to 100 times per minute.
2. Press and knead the Xingjian, Taixi, Sanyinjiao, Xian'gu, Fenglong, and Zusanli acupoints 30 times each, until there is a distending pain in the local area.

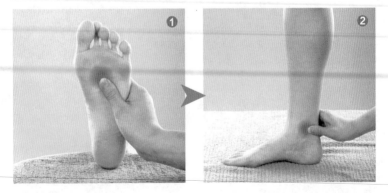

3. Press with thumb tip in turn the reflex zones of the pituitary gland, the cerebellum, the brainstem, the brain (head), and the

neck 20 times each, until there is a distending pain in the local area.

4. Press with thumb tip in turn the reflex zones of the ear, the eye, the liver, the kidney, the adrenal gland, the thyroid gland, and the spleen 20 times each, until there is a distending pain.

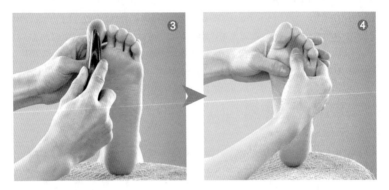

Conclusion: Repeat Step 1, and the treatment is concluded.

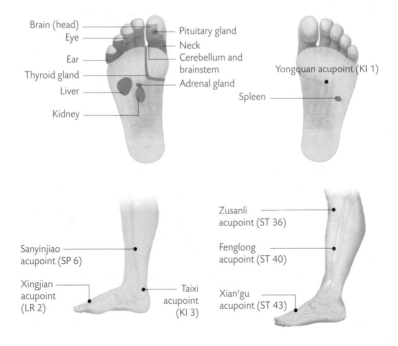

7. Toothaches

To alleviate pain from a toothache, treatment should focus on clearing stomach fire and replenishing kidney yin. Foot reflexology and acupressure can better promote blood circulation to treat inflammation and eliminate pain. It can also strengthen the function of the urinary system and tone the kidneys to remove toxins from the body. In daily life, patients should keep good oral hygiene and brush their teeth in the morning and evening, in proper technique. Exercise your teeth by clicking them 36 times each before getting up in the morning and before going to sleep at night.

Prescription
Do foot reflexology and acupressure two to three times every day. You can repeat the same steps and techniques until the pain stops.

Steps
1. Press with thumb tip in turn the reflex zones of the kidney, the teeth, the stomach and the bladder 100 times each. The level of intensity should be no more than required to generate a distending pain in the local area.
2. From toe to heel, push and press the reflex zone of the ureter 100 times at a rate of 30 to 50 times per minute.
3. From the inner edge to the outside edge of the foot, push and press the reflex zone of the lung and bronchus 50 times each at a rate of 30 to 50 times per minute.

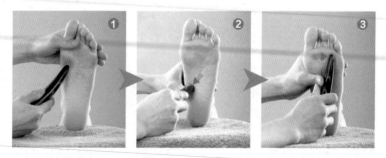

4. Press and knead acupoints such as the Yongquan, Taixi, Neiting, Xian'gu, and Zusanli 30 times each. The level of intensity should

be no more than is necessary to generate a distending pain in the local area.

5. Press with thumb tip the reflex zones of the maxilla, the mandible and the duodenum 50 times each. The intensity of stimulation is no more than necessary to generate a distending pain in the local area.

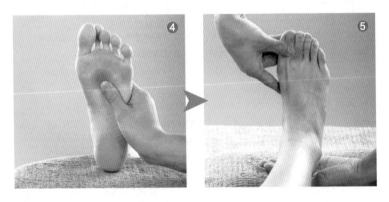

Conclusion: Repeat Steps 1, 2 and 3, decreasing the number of stimulations by half.

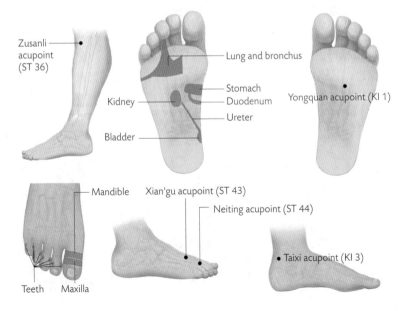

8. Tinnitus

Foot reflexology and acupressure therapy has a certain effect on neurological tinnitus, deafness, and sudden deafness. However, it has little effect on persistent, drug-induced, congenital deafness, or organic deafness of the inner ear. Do not dig the ears, and keep the ear canal clean. Avoid overexertion and fatigue, and limit the frequency of sexual intercourse. All of these precautions will have a positive effect on the treatment and prevention of tinnitus.

Prescription
Do foot reflexology once daily, with 10 sessions forming a full course. Patients with acute onset will need one to two courses of treatment, and long-term foot reflexology treatment is recommended for patients with chronic tinnitus.

In the course of the treatment, patients can do self-massage to enhance the treatment by covering the openings of the external ear channels tightly with both palms while tapping repeatedly on the mastoid area using four fingers, then opening and closing the palms rhythmically over the ear openings. Do this once in the morning and once in the afternoon for 3 to 5 minutes each time.

Steps
1. Press with thumb tip in turn the reflex zones of the kidney and bladder 100 times each until a local distending pain is felt.
2. From toe to heel, push-press the reflex zone to the ureter 100 times at a rate of 30 to 50 times per minute.
3. From the medial side to the lateral side of the foot, push-press

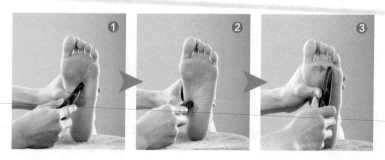

the reflex zone of the lung and bronchus 100 times each, until a local distending pain is felt.

4. Press-knead the Yongquan, Taixi, Zhaohai, Xingjian, Taichong, Yanglingquan, and Zusanli acupoints 30 times each, until a local distending pain is felt.

5. Press with thumb tip the reflex zones for the brain (head), brainstem, trigeminal nerve, ear, liver, gallbladder, lymph nodes of the head and neck region, thoracic lymph node, abdominal lymph node, pelvic lymph node, and solar plexus 50 times each, until a local distending pain is felt.

Conclusion: Repeat Steps 1 through 3, reducing the number of stimulations by half.

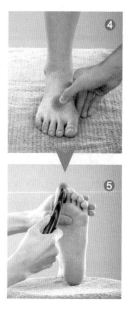

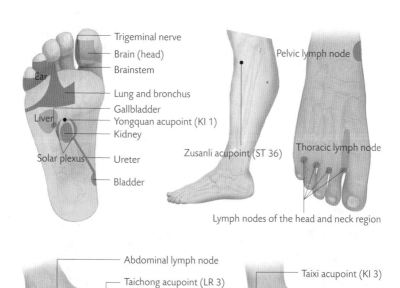

Trigeminal nerve
Brain (head)
Brainstem
Ear
Lung and bronchus
Gallbladder
Liver
Yongquan acupoint (KI 1)
Kidney
Solar plexus
Ureter
Bladder

Pelvic lymph node
Zusanli acupoint (ST 36)
Thoracic lymph node
Lymph nodes of the head and neck region

Abdominal lymph node
Taichong acupoint (LR 3)
Xingjian acupoint (LR 2)

Taixi acupoint (KI 3)
Zhaohai acupoint (KI 6)

9. Common Colds

Massaging acupoints and reflex zones on the feet can not only strengthen the human immune function, but also boost a diversity of physiological functions of the human body, so that the body can exercise its own power of disease resistance and combat infections caused by viruses and bacteria in order to heal ailments. This is a unique characteristic that purely medical treatment does not have.

During the treatment, patients should rest more and drink plenty of water. When there is much soreness in the muscles, pressing and kneading the sore points will effectively alleviate the symptoms.

Prescription
Do foot reflexology twice daily. The patient should feel slightly sweaty but comfortable after each foot reflexology treatment. Avoid copious amounts of sweats. After each foot reflexology session, cover the patient with a blanket to keep warm and avoid repeated attacks of cold-wind.

Steps
1. Press with thumb tip in turn the reflex zones of the kidney and adrenal gland 100 times each. Press towards the heel until a slight local soreness or pain is felt.
2. From toe to heel, push-press the reflex zone of the ureter 50 times. Do this with an even force at a rate of 30 to 50 times per minute. Avoid applying too much pressure. Push-press until a local soreness and distention is felt.
3. Press with thumb tip the reflex zones of the bladder, nose, and lymph nodes of the head and neck region 50 times each, until a slight local soreness and pain is felt.

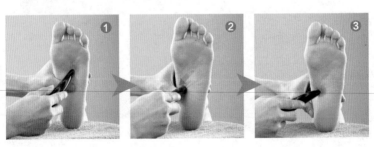

4. From the lateral side to the medial side of the foot, push-press the reflex zone of the lung and bronchus 50 times each, until a local soreness and distention is felt.
5. Press with thumb tip the reflex zones of the thoracic lymph node and throat until a local soreness and distention is felt.
6. Press-knead in turn the Jinmen, Shenmai, Zutonggu, Jinggu and Gongsun acupoints, 30 times each. If the patient has a sore throat, add massages to the Yinbai, Lidui and Bafeng acupoints. Press-knead each point 20 times.

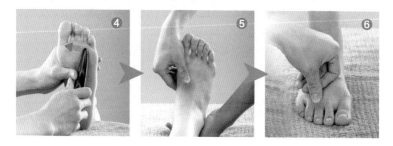

Conclusion: Repeat Steps 1 and 2, reducing the number of stimulations by half.

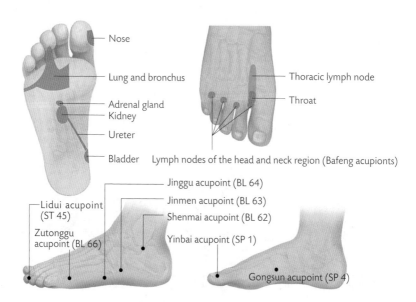

10. Chronic Bronchitis

Chronic bronchitis is mostly related to functional disharmony of such internal organs as the lung, bronchus, spleen, kidney, and liver. Invasion of external evils such as wind and cold is another factor that leads to the acute onset or the exacerbation of chronic bronchitis. The treatment of chronic bronchitis should, therefore, aim to enhance the patient's physical constitution, improve the body's immune system, and regulate the function of the viscera.

In addition to doing foot reflexology treatment, the patient must also lead a regular life, stay warm, and quit smoking and alcohol. His or her accommodations should be quiet and clean, with ample fresh air. Do not live in a damp and dark place.

Prescription

Do foot reflexology twice daily, once in the morning and once in the afternoon, allowing one month for a full course. When the symptoms have subsided, the patient should continue doing foot reflexology at least once daily, accompanied by appropriate exercise.

Steps

1. Press with thumb tip in turn the reflex zones of the kidney, adrenal gland, and bladder 10 times each. The application of pressure can be intensified until a local ache or soreness is felt.
2. From toe to heel, push-press the reflex zone to the ureter 50 times. Both the application of pressure and the speed of stimulation should be even, at a rate of 30 to 50 times per minute.

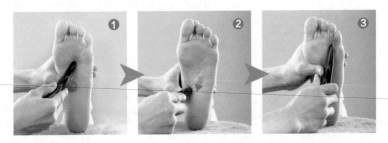

3. Press with thumb tip in turn the reflex zones of the lung, bronchus, thoracic lymph node, tonsil and parathyroid gland 5 times each, until a local ache and soreness is felt.

4. Press with thumb tip in turn the reflex zones of the heart, liver, spleen, stomach and nose 5 times each, until a local ache and soreness is felt.

5. Press-knead the Fenglong, Zusanli, Sanyinjiao, Taichong and Yongquan acupoints 10 times each, until a local ache and soreness is felt.

Conclusion: Repeat Steps 1 and 2, reducing the frequency of stimulations by half to end the treatment.

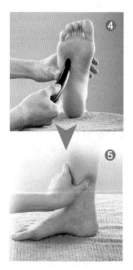

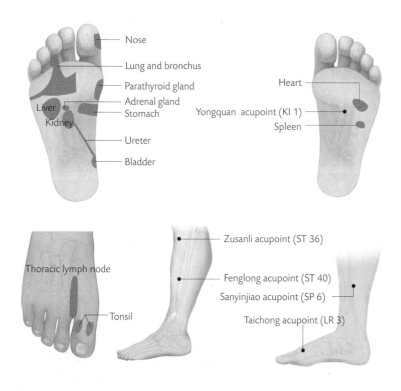

Nose

Lung and bronchus

Parathyroid gland

Heart

Liver

Adrenal gland

Stomach

Kidney

Yongquan acupoint (KI 1)

Spleen

Ureter

Bladder

Thoracic lymph node

Zusanli acupoint (ST 36)

Fenglong acupoint (ST 40)

Sanyinjiao acupoint (SP 6)

Tonsil

Taichong acupoint (LR 3)

11. Asthma

For patients with chronic asthma, perseverance in the massage treatment is recommended. If preventive treatment is done before any seasonal change, the onset of the acute disease can be prevented and the severity reduced. The frequency of asthma attacks can also be decreased.

Patients should actively engage in physical exercise to improve their physical condition. They should also prevent cold and avoid excessive fatigue. Those with a history of allergies should seek to identify the allergens and avoid the intake of those allergens through inhalation, physical contact, or ingestion. A generally light diet is recommended. They should quit smoking and alcohol, and be watchful of seafood intake such as fish, shrimp, and crab, which are likely to trigger allergy and the onset of the disease.

Prescription
Do foot reflexology once daily. Long-term treatment is advised. Increase the number of treatments at the turn of the seasons to twice daily, once in the morning and once in the evening.

Steps
1. Press with thumb tip in turn the reflex zones of the kidney, adrenal gland, pituitary gland and bladder 100 times each until a local distention and pain is felt.
2. From toe to heel, push-press the reflex zone to the ureter 100 times at a rate of 30 to 50 times per minute.
3. From the medial side to the lateral side of the foot, push-press the reflex zone of the lung and bronchus 100 times, at a rate of 30 to 50 times per minute.

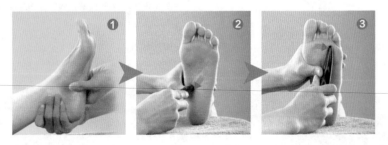

4. Push-knead the Yongquan, Taixi, Zusanli, Fenglong, Shangjuxu and Xingjian acupoints 30 times each, until a local distention and pain is felt.
5. Press with thumb tip the reflex zones of the nose, lymph nodes of the head and neck region, thoracic lymph node, abdominal lymph node and pelvic lymph node 100 times each, until a local distention and pain is felt.
6. From heel to toe, push-press the reflex zone of the ascending colon 50 times. From right to left, push-press the transverse colon 50 times. From toe to heel, push-press the descending colon 50 times. From the lateral side of the foot to the medial side, push-press the reflex zones of the sigmoid colon and rectum 50 times each. All these techniques should be done in the sequence as listed, at a rate of 30 to 50 times per minute.

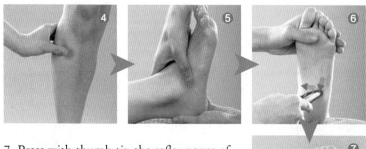

7. Press with thumb tip the reflex zones of the cervical spine, thoracic spine, stomach, gallbladder, liver, and spleen 30 times each, until a local distention and pain is felt.

Conclusion: Repeat Steps 1 through 3 to conclude the session.

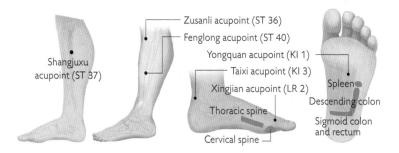

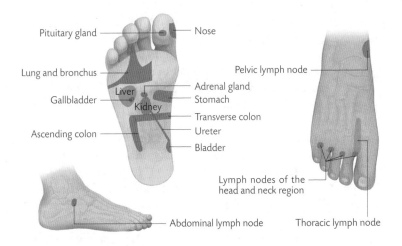

12. Hiccups

This section introduces a general therapeutic method for treating the hiccups through foot reflexology and acupressure. For hiccups caused by other diseases, the additional reflex zones of the kidney, ureter, bladder, lung, and bronchus should be massaged during foot reflexology. Those who are prone to hiccups should refrain from eating cold or spicy foods and maintain a quiet mind. When hiccups occur, patients can direct their focus on doing something else to distract themselves.

Prescription
Common hiccups can be stopped if the following method is used. Some patients, whose hiccups are not stopped after a massage, may extend the duration of foot reflexology to put an end to the hiccups.

Steps
1. Push-press the left foot with force the reflex zones of the diaphragm, stomach and the Zusanli, Neiting and Xian'gu acupoints 20 times each, until a local pain and distention is felt.
2. Do the same with the right foot, following the instructions as specified in Step 1.

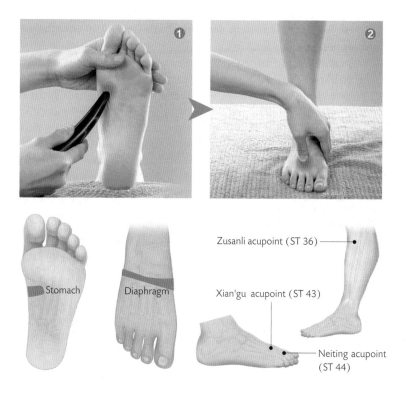

Zusanli acupoint (ST 36)

Stomach   Diaphragm   Xian'gu acupoint (ST 43)

Neiting acupoint (ST 44)

13. Cough

Within 24 hours after the treatment, a cough may deteriorate, and there is an increase in sputum excretion. This is a normal reaction, and the treatment should continue. During the foot reflexology treatment, the patient should maintain a light diet, avoid spicy and pungent foods, and try to quit smoking and consuming alcohol.

Prescription

Acute onset of a cough requires two or three foot reflexology treatments daily. Improvement usually occurs within two or three days. Chronic coughs require one treatment daily, allowing ten sessions for a full course of treatment.

Steps

1. From the medial side to the lateral side of the foot, push-press

the reflex zone of the lung and bronchus 40 to 50 times each, using a massage stick.

2. Press with thumb tip the reflex zones of the throat and bronchus in the direction away from the lower leg 40 to 50 times each.

3. Press with thumb tip the reflex zone of the adrenal gland 80 to 100 times.

4. Using two fingers, push-knead upward toward the lower leg the reflex zone of the tonsil 40 to 50 times.

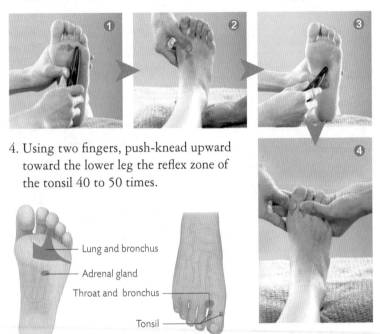

Lung and bronchus

Adrenal gland

Throat and bronchus

Tonsil

14. Chronic Pharyngitis

Foot reflexology works well to coordinate the functions of the viscera, improve the blood circulation of the pharynx, and eliminate inflammation of the pharynx to relieve pain and enhance the body's resistance to the disease.

Patients should avoid spicy and pungent foods during the foot reflexology treatment. They are advised to quit smoking and drinking alcohol, and to empty the bowels regularly. They should maintain a regular lifestyle and do exercises to enhance their physical fitness and prevent common cold. They should wear a facial mask to avoid the inhalation of dusts in the air.

Prescription

Do foot reflexology once daily, allowing 10 sessions for a course of treatment. In the meantime, take appropriate medication to enhance the effects of the treatment.

Steps

1. Press with thumb tip in turn the reflex zones of the kidney, tonsil, throat, bronchus and bladder 100 times each, until a local pain and distention is felt.
2. From toe to heel, push-press the reflex zone to the ureter 100 times at a rate of 30 to 50 times per minute.
3. From the medial side to the lateral side of the foot, push-press the reflex zone of the lung and bronchus 100 times, at a rate of 30 to 50 times per minute.

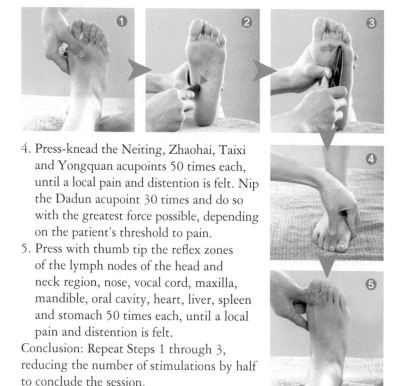

4. Press-knead the Neiting, Zhaohai, Taixi and Yongquan acupoints 50 times each, until a local pain and distention is felt. Nip the Dadun acupoint 30 times and do so with the greatest force possible, depending on the patient's threshold to pain.
5. Press with thumb tip the reflex zones of the lymph nodes of the head and neck region, nose, vocal cord, maxilla, mandible, oral cavity, heart, liver, spleen and stomach 50 times each, until a local pain and distention is felt.

Conclusion: Repeat Steps 1 through 3, reducing the number of stimulations by half to conclude the session.

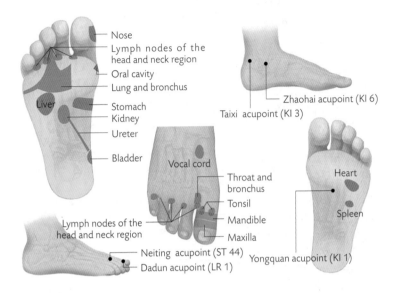

Nose
Lymph nodes of the head and neck region
Oral cavity
Lung and bronchus
Liver
Stomach
Kidney
Ureter
Bladder

Taixi acupoint (KI 3)
Zhaohai acupoint (KI 6)

Vocal cord
Throat and bronchus
Tonsil
Mandible
Maxilla
Lymph nodes of the head and neck region
Heart
Spleen

Neiting acupoint (ST 44)
Dadun acupoint (LR 1)
Yongquan acupoint (KI 1)

15. Chronic Rhinitis

The normal functions of the nose depend mainly on the workings of the lungs and bronchi, as traditional Chinese medicine believes that "the nose is the opening to the lungs and the bronchi." Foot reflexology can disseminate the lung qi and loosen the chest, clearing heat and reducing inflammation, and thus enhancing the ability of the nose to resist disease. Patients should do appropriate outdoor exercise to strengthen their physical fitness. Pay attention to dietary nutrition, eat more vitamin-rich foods, and empty the bowel regularly.

Prescription
Do foot reflexology once daily, allowing a month for a course of treatment. Chronic rhinitis requires long-term, uninterrupted foot reflexology treatment.

Steps
1. From the medial side to the lateral side of the foot, push-press the reflex zone of the lung and bronchus 200 times, at a rate of 30 to 50 times per minute.

2. Press with thumb tip in turn the reflex zones of the nose, kidney and bladder 100 times each until a local pain and distention is felt.
3. From toe to heel, push-press the reflex zone of the ureter 100 times, at a rate of 30 to 50 times per minute.

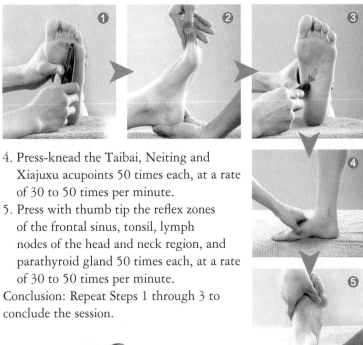

4. Press-knead the Taibai, Neiting and Xiajuxu acupoints 50 times each, at a rate of 30 to 50 times per minute.
5. Press with thumb tip the reflex zones of the frontal sinus, tonsil, lymph nodes of the head and neck region, and parathyroid gland 50 times each, at a rate of 30 to 50 times per minute.

Conclusion: Repeat Steps 1 through 3 to conclude the session.

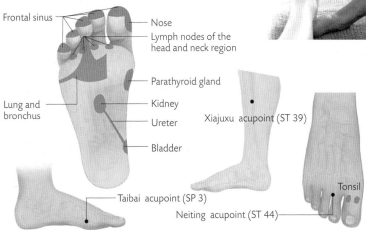

16. Chronic Stomach Disease

Chronic stomach disease is closely related to the liver and spleen. Cold weather, an unhealthy diet, and emotional stress are important triggers of such diseases. Foot reflexology treats the disease by regulating the functions of the stomach, spleen, and liver. However, severe cases of gastric ulcer and duodenal ulcers should not be treated with foot reflexology.

Prescription
Do foot reflexology once daily, allowing ten sessions for a course of treatment. When improvement is evident after a course of treatment, reduce the number of session to once every other day. After a month, further reduce it to twice every week until the symptoms disappear completely. Continue foot reflexology for a month or two to enhance the result.

Steps
1. Press with thumb tip in turn the reflex zones of the stomach, duodenum, spleen, liver, kidney, and bladder 100 times each until local pain and distention is felt.
2. From toe to heel, push-press the reflex zone of the ureter 100 times at a rate of 30 to 50 times per minute.
3. From the medial side to the lateral side of the foot, push-press the reflex zone of the lung and bronchus 100 times, at a rate of 30 to 50 times per minute.

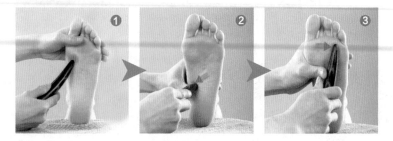

4. Press-knead the Shangjuxu, Xiajuxu, Sanyinjiao, Taichong and Yanglingquan acupoints 30 times each, until local pain and distention is felt.

5. Press with thumb tip the reflex zones of the brain (head), pituitary gland, esophagus, trachea, small intestine and gallbladder 50 times each, until local pain and distention is felt.
6. From heel to toe, push-press the reflex zone to the ascending colon 50 times. From right to left, push-press the reflex zone to the transverse colon 50 times. From toe to heel, push-press the reflex zone to the descending colon 50 times. From the lateral side of the foot to the medial side, push-press the reflex zone to the sigmoid colon and rectum 50 times each, following this sequence at a rate of 30 to 50 times per minute.

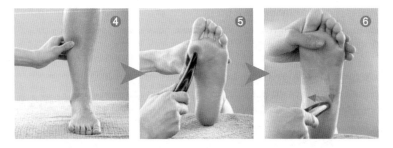

Conclusion: Repeat Steps 1 through 3, reducing the number of stimulations by half to conclude the session.

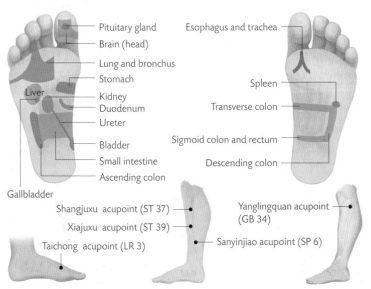

Pituitary gland
Brain (head)
Lung and bronchus
Stomach
Liver
Kidney
Duodenum
Ureter
Bladder
Small intestine
Ascending colon
Gallbladder

Esophagus and trachea
Spleen
Transverse colon
Sigmoid colon and rectum
Descending colon

Shangjuxu acupoint (ST 37)
Xiajuxu acupoint (ST 39)
Taichong acupoint (LR 3)

Yanglingquan acupoint (GB 34)
Sanyinjiao acupoint (SP 6)

17. Psychogenic Vomiting

Psychogenic vomiting is more common in women. The onset is often associated with mental factors and accompanied by other symptoms of neurosis. Typically, patients vomit right after eating. Most patients have a long history of postprandial vomiting. In rare severe cases, patients can experience dehydration, weight loss and malnutrition.

After vomiting stops, it is advised that the patients eat foods that are easy to digest and eat more meals with smaller portions. Patients should maintain a proper diet, avoid binge drinking and eating, and refrain from foods that are heavy, raw, sour, and spicy.

Prescription
Do foot reflexology twice daily. When symptoms have improved, reduce treatment to once daily. When the symptoms disappear completely, do it once every other day, continuing the foot reflexology treatment for a month to enhance the results.

Steps
1. Push-knead in turn the reflex zones of the kidney, adrenal gland, pituitary gland, brain (head), and neck 100 times. The force is on generating a soreness and pain in the local area.
2. From toe to heel, push-press the reflex zone of small intestine 50 times. The operation should be swift, even, rhythmic, and with moderate force.
3. Press with thumb tip the reflex zones of the liver and gallbladder 30 times each. The force is no greater than required to generate a soreness and pain in the local area.

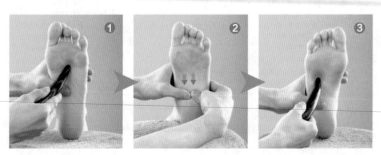

4. Press-knead the Zusanli, Xian'gu, Yongquan, Taichong, and Yanglingquan acupoints until a local soreness and distention is felt.
Conclusion: Repeat Step 1 to complete the session.

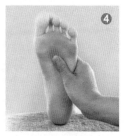

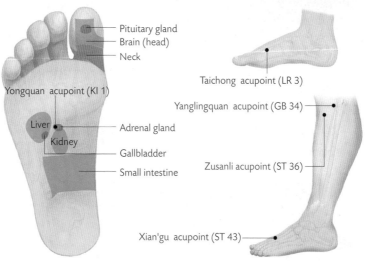

Pituitary gland
Brain (head)
Neck

Yongquan acupoint (KI 1)

Liver
Kidney
Adrenal gland
Gallbladder
Small intestine

Taichong acupoint (LR 3)

Yanglingquan acupoint (GB 34)

Zusanli acupoint (ST 36)

Xian'gu acupoint (ST 43)

18. Diarrhea

Diarrhea is caused by dysfunction of the spleen, stomach, and the large and small intestines. Foot reflexology treatment of chronic diarrhea should follow the principle of reinforcing the spleen and regulating the stomach, warming the kidney and toning the yang, dredging the liver, and regulating qi. With the onset of diarrhea, do not eat carbon hydrates and fatty foods and avoid all raw, cold, and irritating or indigestible foods. Patients should keep warm and avoid overexertion while maintaining a regular diet and lifestyle. The patient should rub his or her abdomen 100 times counterclockwise with the palm every morning and evening.

Prescription

Do foot reflexology once daily, allowing ten sessions for a course of treatment. Take two to four courses for a full treatment. When stool takes shape, continue for one or two more courses to enhance the results, and then reduce to one session every other day. The number of stimulations is also reduced by half at this point.

Steps

1. Press with thumb tip the reflex zones of the kidney and bladder 100 times each until a local distention and pain is felt.
2. From toe to heel, push-press the reflex zone of the ureter 100 times at a rate of 30 to 50 times per minute.
3. From the medial side to the lateral side of the foot, push-press the reflex zone of the lung and bronchus 100 times each at a rate of 30 to 50 times per minute.

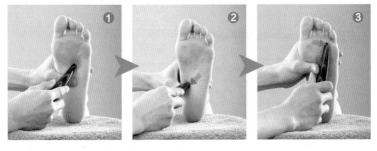

4. Press-knead the reflex zones of the spleen, stomach, and duodenum 100 times each, until a local distention and pain is felt.
5. Press-knead the Shangjuxu, Xiajuxu, Taichong, Taibai and Sanyinjiao acupoints until a local distention and pain is felt.
6. From toe to heel, push-press the reflex zone of the small intestine

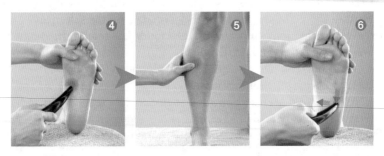

50 times. From heel to toe, push-press the reflex zone to the ascending colon 50 times. From right to left, push-press the reflex zone of the transverse colon 50 times. From toe to heel, push-press the reflex zone of the descending colon 50 times. From the lateral side of the foot to the medial side, push-press the reflex zones of the sigmoid colon and rectum 50 times. Follow this sequence at a rate of 30 to 50 times per minute.

7. Press with thumb tip the reflex zones of the liver, gallbladder, abdominal and pelvic lymph nodes 50 times each, at a rate of 30 to 50 times per minute.

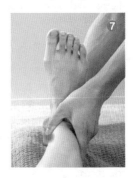

Conclusion: Repeat Steps 1 through 3, reducing the number of stimulations by half to complete the session.

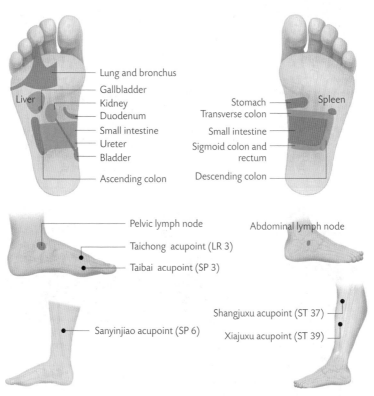

Lung and bronchus

Gallbladder

Liver

Kidney

Duodenum

Small intestine

Ureter

Bladder

Ascending colon

Stomach

Spleen

Transverse colon

Small intestine

Sigmoid colon and rectum

Descending colon

Pelvic lymph node

Abdominal lymph node

Taichong acupoint (LR 3)

Taibai acupoint (SP 3)

Sanyinjiao acupoint (SP 6)

Shangjuxu acupoint (ST 37)

Xiajuxu acupoint (ST 39)

19. Constipation

Patients are advised to eat more fiber-rich foods and empty the
bowels regularly. If constipation appears to be a symptom of other
diseases, the patient should go to the hospital and actively engage
in treating the primary disease, using foot reflexology as an auxiliary
method.

Prescription
It takes only two or three sessions to see improvement when the
constipation is not severe. For severe constipation, however, do foot
reflexology once each morning and once each evening, allowing a
month for a full course of treatment. When the symptoms have
improved, continue to do it once daily before bedtime to enhance
the results.

Steps
1. Press with thumb tip in turn the reflex zones of the stomach,
   duodenum, spleen, liver, kidney and bladder 100 times each
   until a local distention and pain is felt.
2. From toe to heel, push-press the reflex zone of the ureter
   100 times at a rate of 30 to 50 times per minute.
3. From the medial side to the lateral side of the foot, push-press
   the reflex zone of the lung and bronchus 100 times, at a rate of
   30 to 50 times per minute.

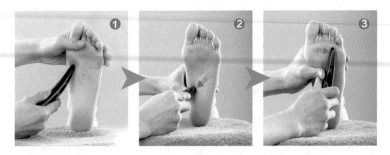

4. Press-knead the Zusanli, Shangjuxu, Xiajuxu, Sanyinjiao,
   Taichong and Yanglingquan acupoints 30 times each, until a
   local distention and pain is felt.

5. Press with thumb tip the reflex zones of the brain (head), pituitary gland, esophagus, trachea, small intestine, and gallbladder 50 times each, until a local distention and pain is felt.

6. From heel to toe, push-press the reflex zone of the ascending colon 50 times. From right to left, push-press the reflex zone of the transverse colon 50 times. From toe to heel, push-press the reflex zone of the descending colon 50 times. From the lateral side of the foot to the medial side, push-press the reflex zones of the sigmoid colon and rectum 50 times. Follow this sequence at a rate of 30 to 50 times per minute.

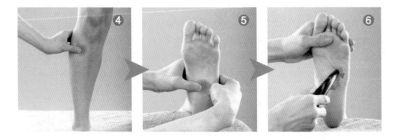

Conclusion: Repeat Steps 1 through 3, reducing the number of stimulations by half to complete the session.

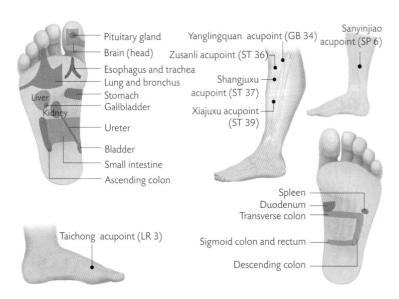

20. Peptic Ulcers

To treat digestive tract ulcers with foot reflexology and acupressure, it is important that patients persevere in the method. Even if symptoms have improved, the treatment should continue for an extended period of time, which is of great significance for enhancing the curative effect and preventing recurrence of the ailment. Attention should be paid to food hygiene. Patients should eat foods easy to digest and in smaller portion for each meal but with more meals. Avoid foods that are pungent and spicy. Quit smoking and drinking alcohol.

After a month or two of foot reflexology treatments, if the condition is aggravated and the patient suddenly loses weight instead of seeing improvement in his or her symptoms, the patient should go to the hospital for examination to rule out the possibility of cancer.

Prescription
Do foot reflexology once daily, allowing ten times for a full course of treatment. If symptoms have improved after two or three courses, do foot reflexology once every other day. When the symptoms have disappeared, continue the foot treatment for one or two more months to enhance the results.

Steps
1. Push-knead the reflex zones of the brain (head) and pituitary gland for two minutes each.
2. Press with thumb tip the reflex zones of the stomach and duodenum 100 times each.
3. Press-knead the reflex zone of the solar plexus, moving clockwise, for two minutes.
4. Press with thumb tip the reflex zone of the abdominal lymph

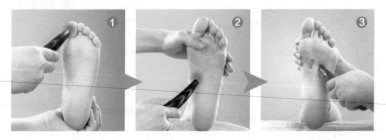

node for 100 times.

5. Knead the reflex zones of the liver, gallbladder, and spleen 100 times each.

6. Press with thumb tip the reflex zones of the adrenal gland and kidney 80 times each.

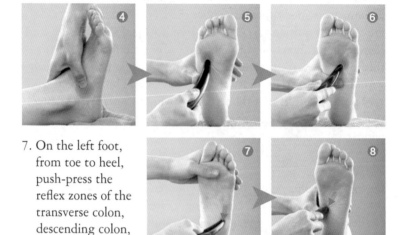

7. On the left foot, from toe to heel, push-press the reflex zones of the transverse colon, descending colon, sigmoid colon, and rectum 60 times

each. On the right foot, from heel to toe, push-press the reflex zones of the ascending colon and transverse colon 60 times each.

8. From toe to heel, push-press the reflex zone of the ureter 80 times. Conclusion: Press with thumb tip the reflex zone of the bladder 80 times.

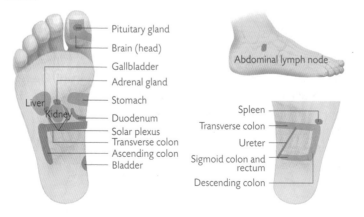

Pituitary gland
Brain (head)
Gallbladder
Adrenal gland
Liver
Kidney
Stomach
Duodenum
Solar plexus
Transverse colon
Ascending colon
Bladder

Abdominal lymph node

Spleen
Transverse colon
Ureter
Sigmoid colon and rectum
Descending colon

21. Inflammation of the Gallbladder and Gallstones

Although gallbladder inflammation (or cholecystitis) and gallstone (or cholelithiasis) can be treated with antibiotics and anti-inflammatory medication to remove the stones, clinical effects are often not satisfactory. Over the past decade, foot reflexology therapy in combination with medication, or even foot reflexology therapy alone, have been used in treating a large number of patients with diseases associated with the gallbladder and biliary tract, with very positive results. For those patients whose stones are no larger than 1.5 cm in diameter, persistent foot reflexology treatment can remove the stones.

Prescription
Do foot reflexology once daily, allowing ten sessions for a full course of treatment. After continuing treatment for two or three courses, reduce by half the number of stimulations in each reflex zone or acupoint if symptoms have shown some improvement. When the symptoms have completely disappeared, continue the foot reflexology treatment to prevent recurrence, but decrease the number of treatment sessions to once every other day. Patients with gallstones should do foot reflexology once daily until the stones are removed, and then reduce the number of treatments by half (once every other day), working 10 to 20 times to enhance the results achieved.

Steps
1. Press with thumb tip in turn the reflex zones of the kidney, bladder, gallbladder, liver, stomach, and duodenum 100 times each until a local pain and distention is felt.
2. From toe to heel, push-press the reflex zone of the ureter 100 times at a rate of 30 to 50 times per minute.
3. From the medial side to the lateral side of the foot, push-press the reflex zone of the lung and bronchus 50 times at a rate of 30 to 50 times per minute.

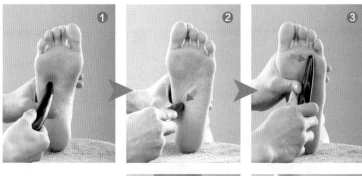

4. Press-knead the Yanglingquan, Dannang, Qiuxu, Taichong and Zusanli acupoints 50 times each, until a local pain and distention is felt.

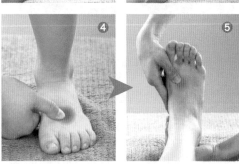

5. Press with thumb tip the reflex zones of the thoracic lymph node, abdominal lymph node, pelvic lymph node, solar plexus and thoracic spine 50 times each, until a local pain and distention is felt.

Conclusion: Repeat Steps 1 through 3, reducing the number of stimulations by half to complete the treatment.

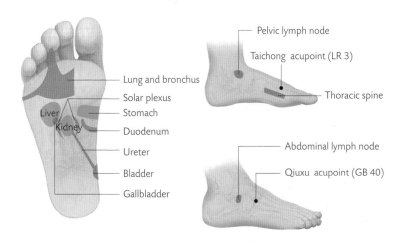

Lung and bronchus
Solar plexus
Liver
Stomach
Kidney
Duodenum
Ureter
Bladder
Gallbladder

Pelvic lymph node
Taichong acupoint (LR 3)
Thoracic spine

Abdominal lymph node
Qiuxu acupoint (GB 40)

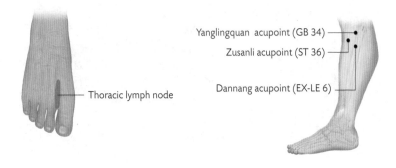

Yanglingquan acupoint (GB 34)

Zusanli acupoint (ST 36)

Dannang acupoint (EX-LE 6)

Thoracic lymph node

22. Chronic Hepatitis and Liver Cirrhosis

In traditional Chinese medicine, chronic hepatitis and cirrhosis both belong in the category of "jaundice" and should be treated primarily by medication. Foot reflexology can be used as an auxiliary treatment to protect and sustain liver function and improve the clinical symptoms.

The liver needs adequate nutrition, so make an effort to take adequate protein, fat, and carbonhydrates but avoid too much animal fat. If the liver function evidently deteriorates, the patient should strictly restrict protein intake. Instead, take plenty of vitamins, of which Vitamin B can effectively prevent the development of a fatty liver and protect and sustain the function of the liver. In addition, Vitamin C promotes metabolism and detoxification, and Vitamin E has an anti-hepatic necrosis effect.

Prescription

Do foot reflexology once daily, allowing three months for a course of treatment. As chronic hepatitis and cirrhosis are both chronic conditions, foot reflexology has to be performed uninterrupted for a long period.

Steps

1. Press with thumb tip in turn the reflex zones of the kidney, liver and bladder 100 times each until a local distention and pain is felt.
2. From toe to heel, push-press the reflex zone of the ureter 100 times at a rate of 30 to 50 times per minute.

3. From the medial side to the lateral side of the foot, push-press the reflex zone of the lung and bronchus 100 times, at a rate of 30 to 50 times per minute.

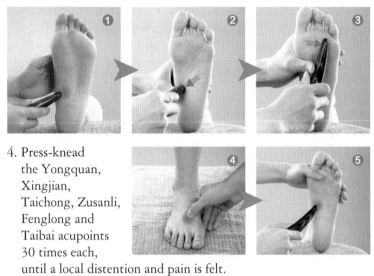

4. Press-knead the Yongquan, Xingjian, Taichong, Zusanli, Fenglong and Taibai acupoints 30 times each, until a local distention and pain is felt.

5. Press with thumb tip the reflex zones of the gallbladder, stomach, duodenum, thoracic spine, solar plexus, and parathyroid gland 50 times each, until a local distention and pain is felt.

Conclusion: Repeat Steps 1 through 3 to complete the session.

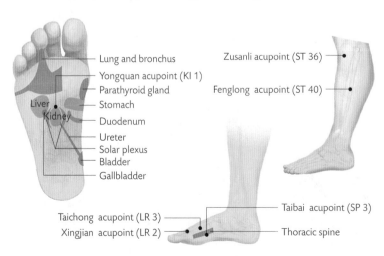

Lung and bronchus
Yongquan acupoint (KI 1)
Parathyroid gland
Liver
Kidney
Stomach
Duodenum
Ureter
Solar plexus
Bladder
Gallbladder

Zusanli acupoint (ST 36)
Fenglong acupoint (ST 40)

Taibai acupoint (SP 3)

Taichong acupoint (LR 3)
Xingjian acupoint (LR 2)
Thoracic spine

23. Chronic Nephritis

Traditional Chinese medicine holds that this disease is categorized as "edema." From the clinical dialectical perspective of TCM, it is often the result of yang deficiency in the spleen and kidneys. Therefore, foot reflexology therapy mainly focuses on reinvigorating the spleen and toning the kidneys in order to facilitate the removal of water and eliminate swelling. By stimulating the acupoints connected to the related organs, the excretion of water and metabolic discharge and toxic substances will be enhanced and the function of the immune system will be strengthened.

Patients should lead a regular life and avoid overexertion, making sure they have enough sleep. Avoid wind pathogen, sexual intercourses, smoking, and drinking alcohol. Keep a diet rich in nutrition. For grains, red bean congee and coix seed congee are recommended, while for meat, beef and lean pork are recommended, and for vegetables, winter melon is best.

Prescription
Do foot reflexology continually once a day.

Steps
1. Press with thumb tip in turn the reflex zones of the kidney, adrenal gland and bladder 100 times each until a local distention and pain is felt.
2. From toe to heel, push-press the reflex zone of the ureter 100 times at a rate of 30 to 50 times per minute.
3. From the medial side to the lateral side of the foot, push-press the reflex zone of the lung and bronchus 100 times, at a rate of 30 to 50 times per minute.

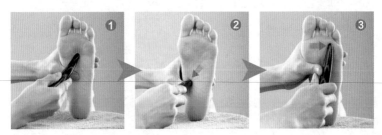

4. Press-knead the Yongquan, Taixi, Sanyinjiao, Taichong, Neiting and Zusanli acupoints 50 times each, until a local distention and pain is felt.

5. From heel to toe, push-press the reflex zone to the thyroid gland 50 times, at a rate of the 30 to 50 times per minute.

6. Press with thumb tip the reflex zones of the spleen, stomach, small intestine, parathyriod gland, gonad 1 (sex gland), brain (head), pituitary gland, solar plexus, abdominal lymph node, pelvic lymph node and blood pressure point 50 times each, until a local distention and pain is felt.

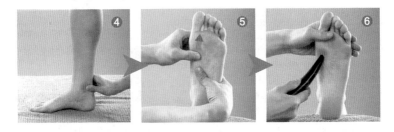

Conclusion: Repeat Steps 1 through 3 to complete the session.

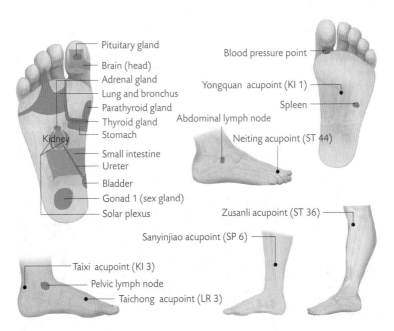

24. Urolithiasis

It is best to treat this disease at the onset of pain, particularly when a patient is experiencing excruciating pain, as this allows for a greater likelihood of removing the stones. When the pain has subsided after treatment, this is often a signal that the stone excretion will begin. For stones in the upper section of the ureter, or if the diameter of the stone is over 1 cm, this indicates that the foot massage treatment has so far proved ineffective, so additional treatments should be considered. Even in conditions suitable for foot reflexology treatment, if severe pain persists or there is blood in the urine, the patient should go to the hospital for immediate treatment.

Patients should drink plenty of water. They should excrete a daily volume of about 2000 ml of urine. They should eat more fruits and vegetables. In the meantime, physical exercise of more vigorous intensity is advised, such as rope skipping, running, mountain climbing, and ball games, which are conducive to the downward journey of the stones, and therefore their excretion.

Prescription
Do foot reflexology once in the morning and once in the evening for ten days.

Steps
1. Press with thumb tip in turn the reflex zones of the kidney and bladder 200 times until a local pain and distention is felt.
2. From toe to heel, push-press the reflex zone of the ureter 200 times at a rate of 30 to 50 times per minute.
3. From the medial side to the lateral side of the foot, push-press the reflex zone of the lung and bronchus 100 times, at a rate of

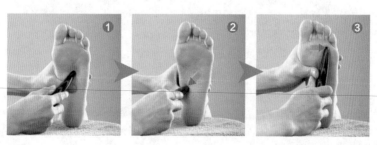

30 to 50 times per minute.

4. Press-knead the Yongquan, Yanglingquan, Yinlingquan, Sanyinjiao, Weizhong, Taixi and Xingjian acupoints 30 times each, until a local pain and distention is felt. Nip-press the Dadun acupoints 10 times.

5. Press with thumb tip the reflex zones of the liver, gallbladder, parathyroid gland, thoracic spine, lumbar spine, abdominal lymph node and pelvic lymph node 50 times each, until a local pain and distention is felt.

6. From heel to toe, push-press the reflex zone of the thyroid gland 50 times, at a rate of 30 to 50 times per minute.

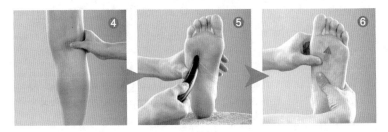

Conclusion: Repeat Steps 1 and 2 to complete the session.

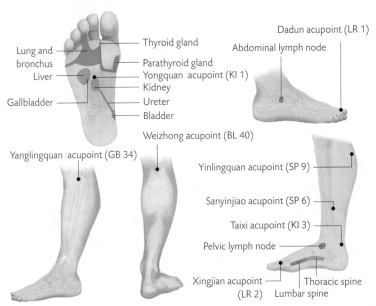

25. Trigeminal Neuralgia

Foot reflexology therapy has proven effecive in the treatment of primary trigeminal neuralgia. Several courses of treatment will usually reduce the frequency of onsets and alleviate the pain associated with the aliment. If patients persevere in the treatment, there is also a chance to cure the disease. For secondary trigeminal neuralgia, foot reflexology is only an auxiliary treatment that aims to relieve pain.

Patients should maintain a positive attitude and avoid mental stress. They should participate in appropriate physical exercise, but avoid overexertion. Do not eat irritating foods and seafoods that are likely to trigger the onset. Avoid alcohol and tobacco.

Prescription
Do foot reflexology twice daily, allowing ten days for a course of treatment. If symptoms have obviously improved after a few courses of treatment, do reflexology once daily until the disease is cured. Do two more courses of treatment to enhance the results and prevent the disease's recurrence.

Steps
1. Press with thumb tip in turn the reflex zones of the trigimenial nerve, brain (head), brainstem, kidney and bladder 50 times each until a local distention and pain is felt.
2. From toe to heel, push-press the reflex zone of the ureter 50 times at a rate of 30 to 50 times per minute.
3. From the medial side to the lateral side of the foot, push-press

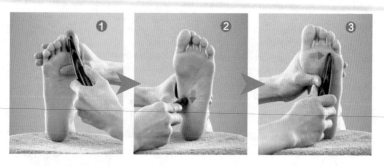

the reflex zone of the lung and bronchus 50 times, at a rate of 30 to 50 times per minute.

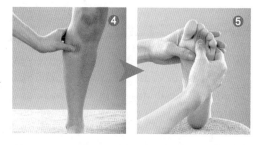

4. Press-knead the Xian'gu, Neiting, Taichong, Xingjian, Yanglingquan, Sanyinjiao and Zusanli acupoints 30 times each, until a local distention and pain is felt.
5. Press with thumb tip the reflex zones of the nose, eye, ear, oral cavity and tooth 30 times each, until a local distention and pain is felt.

Conclusion: Repeat Steps 1 through 3 to complete the session.

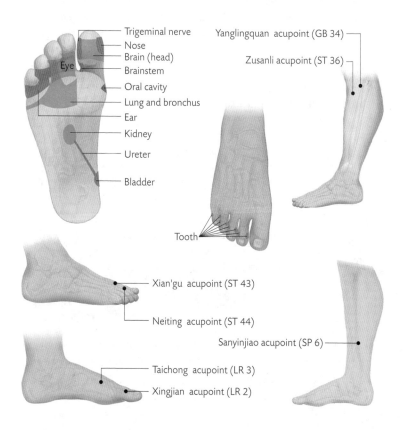

26. Facial Paralysis

Foot reflexology therapy works effectively in the treatment of facial paralysis. In the course of the treatment, patients can hand-massage the affected facial muscles on their own, usually for 5 to 10 minutes at a time. Hot compresses using a towel on the affected area can also be added twice daily for 10 minutes each time. Be careful with the temperature, which should not be so high as to cause burns. In addition, patients should do some exercise to restore related functions of the face during the recovery period. They can practice facial expressions in front of a mirror, starting with knitting the brows, frowning, wrinkling the nose, exposing the teeth, closing the eyes and stretching the ends of their mouths. Such exercise can stifle the development of the disease. If the facial paralysis happens in winter, patients should wear a facial mask when going out to prevent the face from being attacked by cold and wind pathogens.

Prescription
Do foot reflexology once daily for ten sessions as a course of treatment. The treatment usually lasts for three to four courses.

Steps
1. Press with thumb tip the reflex zones of the kidney and bladder 50 times each until a local distension and pain is felt.

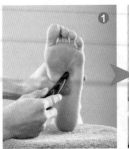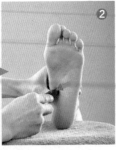

2. From toe to heel, push-press the reflex zone of the ureter 50 times at a rate of 30 to 50 times per minute.
3. From the medial side to the lateral side of the foot, push-press the reflex zone of the lung and bronchus 50 times each, at a rate of 30 to 50 times per minute.
4. Press-knead the Yanglingquan, Zusanli and Xian'gu acupoints

50 times each, until a local distension and pain is felt.

5. Press with thumb tip the reflex zones of the brain (head), neck, maxilla, mandible, nose, eye, ear and lymph nodes of the head and neck region 100 times each, until a local distension and pain is felt.

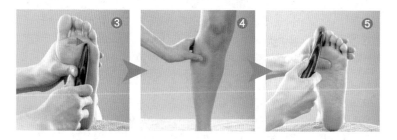

Conclusion: Repeat Steps 1 through 3 to complete the session.

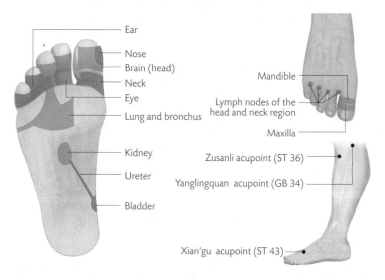

27. Neurodermatitis

Foot reflexology therapy can facilitate the flow of lung qi to relieve chest stuffiness, clear heat, remove dampness, sooth the liver, tranquilize the heart, and calm the mind, thus achieving the effect of alleviating itching. Foot reflexology can also regulate the functional activities of the cerebral cortex and nervous system. Through regulation of the nerve and body fluid, the body will adapt to changes in the internal and external environment and maintain the normal function of the whole body.

During the treatment, patients should avoid scratching, rubbing, or using hot water to alleviate itching. They are advised to actively treat other sources of the infection. Avoid drinking alcohol, strong tea, or eating spicy and pungent foods. Lead a regular life, maintain a balanced emotional state and get plenty of sleep.

Prescription

Do foot reflexology once daily for ten sessions as a course of treatment. Most patients will find decreased severity of itching after three or four courses. Continue with the same foot reflexology until subjective feelings of itching have disappeared, then reduce the number of treatments to once every other day until the skin is completely restored to the smoothness. This disease is likely to recur, so it is better to continue treatment long term.

Steps

1. Press with thumb tip in turn the reflex zones of the kidney and bladder 50 times each until a local pain and distention is felt.
2. From toe to heel, push-press the reflex zone of the ureter 50 times at a rate of 30 to 50 times per minute.
3. From the medial side to the lateral side of the foot, push-press the reflex zone of the lung and bronchus 100 times each, at a rate of 30 to 50 times per minute.
4. Press-knead the Xiajuxu, Taichong, Xingjian, Yongquan and Zusanli acupoints 50 times each, until a local pain and distention is felt.

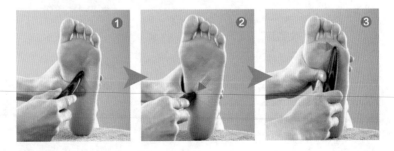

5. Press with thumb tip the reflex zones of the brain (head), heart, liver, adrenal gland, pituitary gland and insomnia point 100 times each, until a local pain and distention is felt.

6. From heel to toe, push-press the reflex zone of the ascending colon 50 times. From right to left, push-press the reflex zone of the transverse colon 50 times. From toe to heel, push-press the reflex zone of the descending colon 50 times. From the lateral side of the foot to the medial side, push-press the reflex zones of the sigmoid colon and rectum 50 times each. Follow this sequence at a rate of 30 to 50 times per minute.

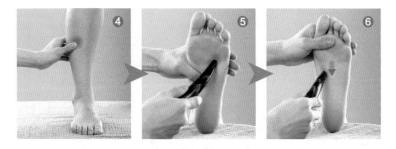

Conclusion: Repeat Steps 1 through 3 to conclude the session.

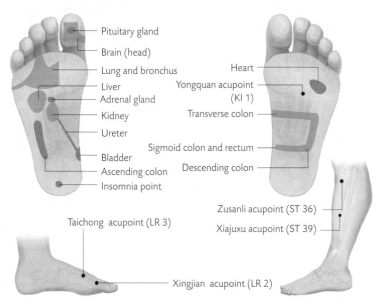

28. Stroke Sequelae

Foot reflexology must be performed after the acute phase of
this illness has passed. Therapeutic exercise of the joint during
treatment is beneficial to the improvement of the state of paralysis.
For people with reduced mobility, their positions should be changed
regularly, or the suppressed area be massaged or squeeze-pinched to
prevent bedsores. Attention should be paid to diet, and they should
keep a regular life and maintain a positive mood. Make sure that
the treatment is correct and uninterrupted.

Prescription
Do foot reflexology once daily. Continued treatment of three
months makes a full course of treatment. Most patients will need
three to four courses. Apply stronger force when stimulating the
affected side.

Steps
1. Press with thumb tip the reflex zones of the kidney, adrenal
   gland and bladder until a local distention and pain is felt.
2. From toe to heel, push-press the reflex zone of the ureter
   100 times at a rate of 30 to 50 times per minute.
3. From the medial side to the lateral side of the foot, push-press
   the reflex zone of the lung and bronchus 100 times each at a rate
   of 30 to 50 times per minute.

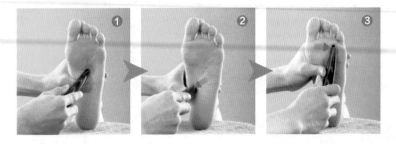

4. Press-knead the Zusanli, Jiexi, Sanyinjiao, Taixi, Yongquan,
   Taichong, Yanglingquan, Shenmai and Zhaohai acupoints
   30 times each, until a local distention and pain is felt.

5. Press with thumb tip the reflex zones of the brain (head), pituitary gland, organ of balance, spleen, stomach and a diversity of lymph nodes 50 times each, until a local distention and pain is felt.

6. Push-press the reflex zones of the small intestine, ascending colon, transverse colon, descending colon, sigmoid colon and rectum at a rate of 30 to 50 times per minute.

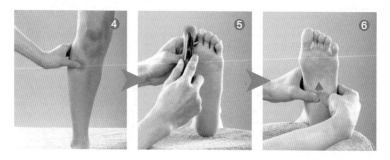

7. Press with thumb tip the reflex zones of the shoulder, elbow joint, knee joint and hip joint 30 times each.

8. Push-press in turn the reflex zones of the cervical spine, thoracic spine, lumbar spine, sacrum, inner coccyx and outer coccyx. Push-press one reflex zone to the next in the sequence until all the reflex zones are stimulated, and this is considered once, do this 30 times.

9. From heel to toe, push-press the reflex zone of the thyroid gland 50 times, at a rate of 30 to 50 times per minute.

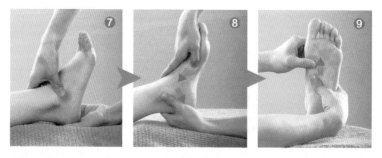

Conclusion: Repeat Steps 1 through 3, reducing the number of stimulations by half to complete the session.

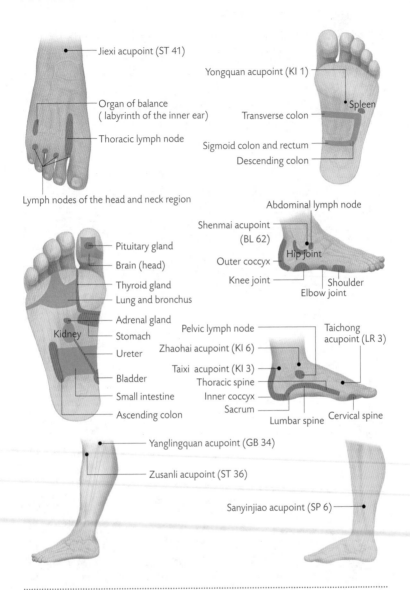

Jiexi acupoint (ST 41)

Organ of balance
(labyrinth of the inner ear)

Thoracic lymph node

Lymph nodes of the head and neck region

Yongquan acupoint (KI 1)

Spleen

Transverse colon

Sigmoid colon and rectum

Descending colon

Pituitary gland

Brain (head)

Thyroid gland

Lung and bronchus

Adrenal gland

Kidney — Stomach

Ureter

Bladder

Small intestine

Ascending colon

Abdominal lymph node

Shenmai acupoint
(BL 62)

Outer coccyx

Knee joint

Hip joint

Shoulder

Elbow joint

Pelvic lymph node

Zhaohai acupoint (KI 6)

Taixi acupoint (KI 3)

Thoracic spine

Inner coccyx

Sacrum

Lumbar spine

Taichong
acupoint (LR 3)

Cervical spine

Yanglingquan acupoint (GB 34)

Zusanli acupoint (ST 36)

Sanyinjiao acupoint (SP 6)

29. Insomnia

Foot reflexology is used to treat and prevent insomnia mainly through stimulating acupoints connected to the *zangfu* organs and regulating their functions. The kidneys are important excretory organs. When they underperform, some of the water in the body is retained, resulting in edema and insomnia. That is to say that low kidney function is considered one of the main causes of insomnia. Therefore, massaging the acupoints and reflex zones connected to the kidneys is the key to achieving good therapeutic results. Insomnia is usually a chronic process, and therefore it takes a long time before a satisfactory result is achieved.

Prescription

Do foot reflexology once daily, with two weeks making a full course of treatment. If a patient can take his or her own initiative to further continue self-massage, the result will be better. For people with severe insomnia, press the reflex zone of the solar plexus as many as 300 times.

Steps

1. Press with thumb tip in turn the reflex zones of the kidney, adrenal gland, bladder, pituitary gland, gonad 1 (sex gland) and liver 10 times each, with slightly stronger pressure, until a local distention a nd soreness is felt.
2. Push-press the reflex zone of the ureter 50 times in the direction from toe to heel until a local distention and soreness is felt, at a rate of 30 to 50 times per minute.
3. Press with thumb tip in turn the reflex zones of the solar plexus, thyroid gland, parathyroid gland, heart, spleen, stomach, small intestine and insomnia point 30 times each, until a local distention and soreness is felt.

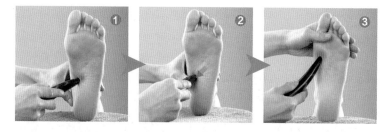

4. Press-knead the Taixi, Taichong and Sanyinjiao acupoints 30 times.
5. Rub the Yongquan acupoint 100 times until a local warm

sensation is felt. While rubbing, breathe naturally without holding the breath. Rub evenly at a rate of 80 to 100 times per minute.

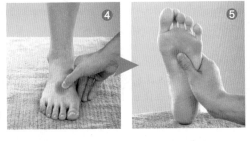

Conclusion: Repeat Steps 1, 2 and 5 to complete the session.

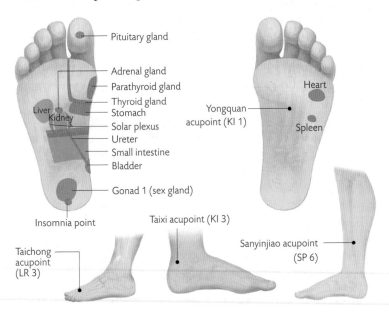

Pituitary gland

Adrenal gland
Parathyroid gland
Thyroid gland
Liver
Kidney
Stomach
Solar plexus
Ureter
Small intestine
Bladder

Heart

Yongquan acupoint (KI 1)

Spleen

Gonad 1 (sex gland)

Insomnia point

Taixi acupoint (KI 3)

Taichong acupoint (LR 3)

Sanyinjiao acupoint (SP 6)

30. Hypersomnia

Foot reflexology can regulate the functions of the *zangfu* organs, mainly through stimulating reflex zones on the foot that are connected to the related organs, thereby achieving the purpose of reinvigorating energy and facilitating awakening. If patients can soak their feet in warm water before going to bed to the point that a warm sensation is felt all over the body, the result will be much more effective. In the course of foot reflexology treatment, patients are advised to actively participate in physical exercise and maintain a positive mood.

Prescription

Do foot reflexology once in the morning and once in the evening for ten sessions to make a full course of treatment. Improvement will usually occur after one or two courses of treatment.

Steps

1. Press with thumb tip the reflex zones of the brain (head) and pituitary gland 60 times each.
2. Press-knead the reflex zone of the kidney for 1 minute.
3. From toe to heel, push-press the reflex zone of the ureter 50 times for about 1 minute.

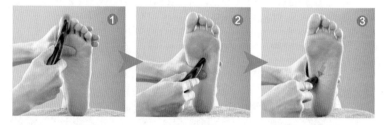

4. Press with thumb tip the reflex zone of the bladder 60 times.
5. From toe to heel, push-press the reflex zone of the thyroid gland 60 times.
6. Press with thumb tip the reflex zone of the parathyroid gland 50 times.

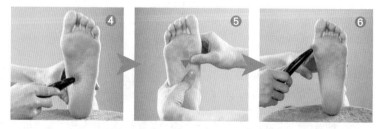

7. From the medial side to the lateral side of the foot, push-press the reflex zone of the lung and bronchus 60 times.
8. Press with thumb tip the reflex zone of the solar plexus clockwise 60 times.
9. Press with thumb tip the reflex zone of the heart 80 times.

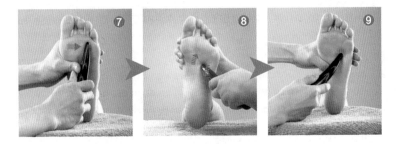

10. Press with thumb tip the reflex zones of the spleen and stomach 100 times.
11. Press with thumb tip the reflex zones of the femoral joint and hip joint 100 times each.
12. Bend the finger and press with thumb tip the reflex zone of the gonad 1 (sex gland) 60 times.

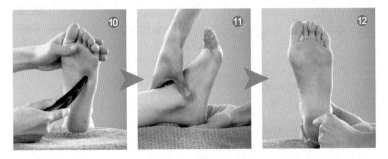

Conclusion: Repeat Steps 2 through 4, reducing the number of stimulations by half to complete the session.

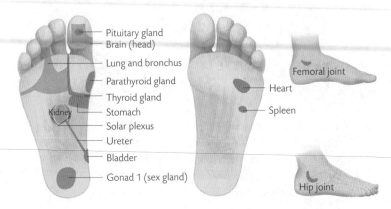

Pituitary gland
Brain (head)
Lung and bronchus
Parathyroid gland
Thyroid gland
Kidney
Stomach
Solar plexus
Ureter
Bladder
Gonad 1 (sex gland)

Heart
Spleen

Femoral joint
Hip joint

31. Night Sweats

Foot reflexology is used to treat and prevent night sweats mainly by nourishing and toning the liver and kidney yin. The kidneys are considered the root of life. In traditional Chinese medicine, the liver and kidneys belong to the lower burner (part of triple burner/ *sanjiao* consisting of upper burner, middle burner, and lower burner). By stimulating the acupoints connected to the liver and kidneys, foot reflexology regulates the functions of the liver and kidneys, thus nourishing yin and alleviating perspiration.

Prescription
Do foot reflexology once or twice daily, continuing for two weeks for a full course of treatment. Depending on the severity of the condition, this can continue for three or four more courses.

Steps
1. Press with thumb tip in turn the reflex zones of the adrenal gland, kidney, bladder, heart and spleen 100 times each until a slight local distention and soreness is felt.
2. Press with thumb tip the reflex zone of the ureter 50 times, from toe to heel, with pressure applied evenly.
3. From the medial side to the lateral side of the foot, push-press the reflex zone of the lung and bronchus 100 times, with pressure applied evenly.

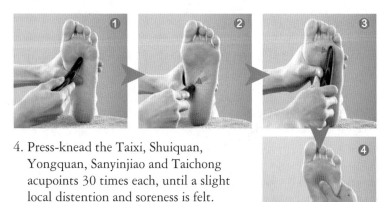

4. Press-knead the Taixi, Shuiquan, Yongquan, Sanyinjiao and Taichong acupoints 30 times each, until a slight local distention and soreness is felt.
Conclusion: Repeat Steps 1 through 3, reducing the number of stimulations by half.

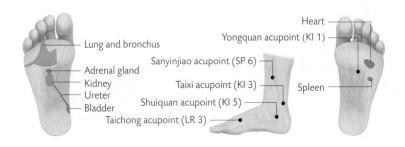

32. Anemia

By stimulating some corresponding acupoints, the functions of the *zangfu* organs are regulated, especially the spleen and stomach, whose main functions are to generate and transform the vital qi and blood, thereby achieving the goal of replenishing qi and toning the blood. In the course of the treatment, patients should pay attention to nutrition intake, eating more foods rich in iron and protein, such as green vegetables, soybeans, eggs, animal liver, and animal blood.

Prescription

Do foot reflexology once daily for three months as a course of treatment. When improvement is evident after a three-month treatment, reduce treatments to once every other day.

Steps

1. Press with thumb tip in turn the reflex zones of the kidney, bladder, spleen, stomach, heart, liver, small intestine and gonad 2 (sex gland) 100 times each until a local distention and pain is felt.
2. From toe to heel, push-press the reflex zones of the ureter and thyroid gland 100 times each at a rate of 30 to 50 times per minute.
3. From the medial side to the lateral side of the foot, push-press the reflex zone of the lung and bronchus 100 times, at a rate of 30 to 50 times per minute.
4. Press-knead the Zusanli, Sanyinjiao, Taixi, Yongquan, Shangjuxu and Xiajuxu acupoints 30 times each, until a local distention and pain is felt.
5. From heel to toe, push-press the reflex zone of the ascending

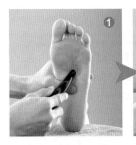
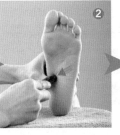
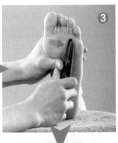
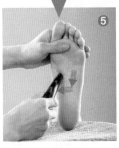

colon. From right to left, push-press the reflex zone of the transverse colon. From toe to heel, push-press the reflex zone of the descending colon. And finally from the lateral side of the foot to the medial side, push-press the reflex zones of the sigmoid colon and rectum, 50 times in total. Press hard and quickly, but move along with ease, until a local distention and pain is felt. For those with hemorrhoids, push-press additionally the reflex zone of the anus 50 times.

Conclusion: Repeat Steps 1 through 3, reducing the number of stimulations by half to conclude the session.

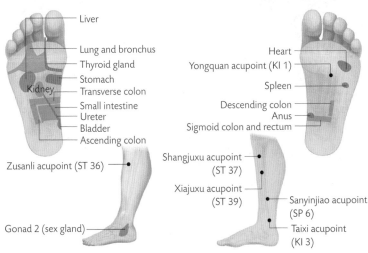

Liver
Lung and bronchus
Thyroid gland
Stomach
Kidney — Transverse colon
Small intestine
Ureter
Bladder
Ascending colon
Zusanli acupoint (ST 36)
Gonad 2 (sex gland)

Heart
Yongquan acupoint (KI 1)
Spleen
Descending colon
Anus
Sigmoid colon and rectum
Shangjuxu acupoint (ST 37)
Xiajuxu acupoint (ST 39)
Sanyinjiao acupoint (SP 6)
Taixi acupoint (KI 3)

33. Obesity

Foot reflexology therapy is effective for weight loss, without causing any harmful side effects. For obesity caused by endocrine disorders, foot reflexology treatment should focus on regulating the endocrine function, thereby regulating fat metabolism in the body. For obesity caused by overeating, it should focus on regulating the function of the gastrointestinal tract and reducing the amount of food intake, thereby reducing the accumulation of fat.

Prescription
Do foot reflexology once daily, allowing one month for a full course of treatment.

Steps
1. Press with thumb tip in turn the reflex zones of the kidney and bladder 100 times until a local distention and pain is felt.
2. From toe to heel, push-press the reflex zone of the ureter 100 times at a rate of 30 to 50 times per minute.
3. From the medial side to the lateral side of the foot, push-press the reflex zone of the lung and bronchus 50 times, at a rate of 30 to 50 times per minute.

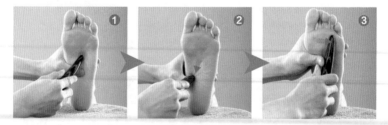

4. Press-knead the Sanyinjiao, Yongquan, Zusanli, Shangjuxu, Xiajuxu and Neiting acupoints 30 times each, until a local distention and pain is felt.
5. Press with thumb tip the reflex zones of the pituitary gland, gonad 1 (sex gland) and adrenal gland 100 times each, until a local distention and pain is felt.
6. From heel to toe, push-press the reflex zone of the thyroid gland 100 times, at a rate of 30 to 50 times per minute.

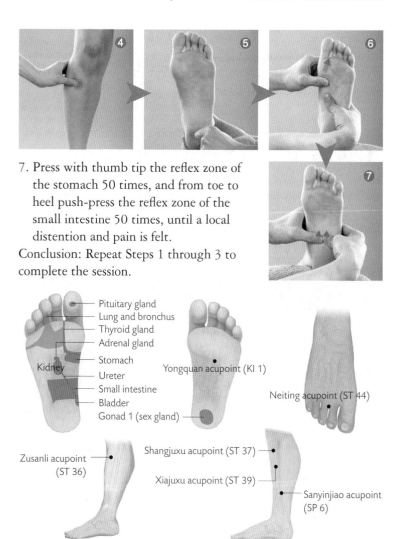

7. Press with thumb tip the reflex zone of the stomach 50 times, and from toe to heel push-press the reflex zone of the small intestine 50 times, until a local distention and pain is felt.

Conclusion: Repeat Steps 1 through 3 to complete the session.

Pituitary gland
Lung and bronchus
Thyroid gland
Adrenal gland
Stomach
Kidney
Ureter
Small intestine
Bladder
Gonad 1 (sex gland)

Yongquan acupoint (KI 1)

Neiting acupoint (ST 44)

Zusanli acupoint (ST 36)

Shangjuxu acupoint (ST 37)
Xiajuxu acupoint (ST 39)
Sanyinjiao acupoint (SP 6)

34. Chronic Open-Angle Glaucoma

The main feature of this disease is elevated intraocular pressure, so close attention should be paid to the changes in pressure around the eye. In the course of foot reflexology treatment, patients should be engaged in some appropriate physical labor and reduce the amount of mental work, while also doing regular physical exercise to the best of their ability and avoiding mental stress.

If emotional factors set off an acute onset and the intraocular pressure rises as high as 45 mm Hg or more, the patient should seek medical treatment from a doctor.

Prescription

Do foot reflexology once daily, allowing ten days for a course of treatment. The intensity of stimulation should be gentle.

Steps

1. Press with thumb tip the reflex zones of the kidney and adrenal gland 100 times each.
2. From toe to heel, push-press the reflex zone of the ureter 100 times.
3. Press with thumb tip the reflex zone of the bladder 100 times.

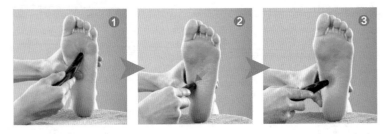

4. From the medial side to the lateral side of the foot, push-press the reflex zone of the lung and bronchus 50 times.
5. Press with thumb tip the reflex zones of the eye, spleen and stomach 100 times each.
6. Press with thumb tip the reflex zones of the brain (head), frontal sinus, neck, liver, gallbladder and lymph nodes of the head and neck region 50 times each.

Conclusion: Repeat Steps 1 through 3, reducing the number of stimulations by half to complete the session.

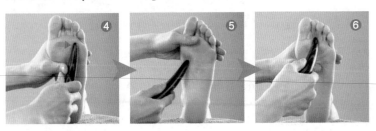

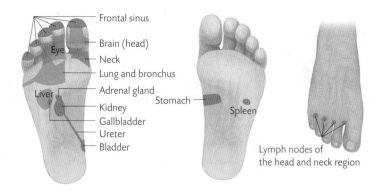

Frontal sinus
Brain (head)
Eye
Neck
Lung and bronchus
Adrenal gland
Liver
Stomach
Kidney
Spleen
Gallbladder
Ureter
Bladder
Lymph nodes of
the head and neck region

35. Locked Shoulder

Foot reflexology is quite effective for treating inflammation
around the shoulder, if combined with some exercise to improve
the mobility of the shoulder. Foot reflexology can improve local
blood circulation, expedite the absorption of discharge, dredge
the meridians, and alleviate the pain, while exercise can loosen the
adhesion and lubricate the joint, thereby expediting the recovery of
the shoulder joints. The two methods complement each other.

During treatment, avoid lifting heavy objects and keep the
affected area warm. Hot compresses can be used as an auxiliary
treatment once daily for ten minutes. Make sure the water
temperature is cool enough to avoid burning the skin.

Prescription
Do foot reflexology once daily, allowing ten sessions for a course of
treatment.

Steps
1. Press with thumb tip in turn the reflex zones of the kidney and
   bladder 50 times each until a local distention and pain is felt.
2. From toe to heel, push-press the reflex zone of the ureter
   50 times at a rate of 30 to 50 times per minute.
3. From the medial side to the lateral side of the foot, push-press
   the reflex zone of the lung and bronchus 50 times, at a rate of
   30 to 50 times per minute.

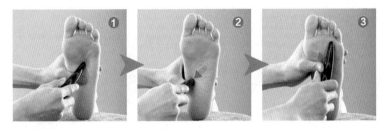

4. Press-knead the Yanglingquan, Xuanzhong, Zusanli and Shenmai acupoints 30 times each, until a local distention and pain is felt.

5. Press with thumb tip the reflex zones of the shoulder, shoulder blade and trapezius 100 times each, until a local distention and pain is felt.

6. Press with thumb tip the reflex zones of the neck, upper arm, cervical spine, thoracic spine, liver and spleen 50 times each, until a local distention and pain is felt.

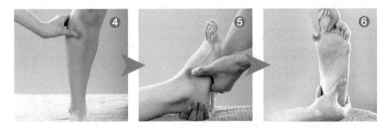

Conclusion: Repeat Steps 1 through 3, reducing the number of stimulations by half to complete the session.

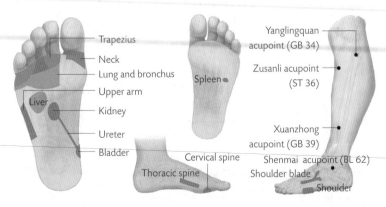

Trapezius
Neck
Lung and bronchus
Upper arm
Liver
Kidney
Ureter
Bladder
Spleen
Cervical spine
Thoracic spine
Yanglingquan acupoint (GB 34)
Zusanli acupoint (ST 36)
Xuanzhong acupoint (GB 39)
Shenmai acupoint (BL 62)
Shoulder blade
Shoulder

36. Cervical Spondylosis

Combined with exercise that help restore the function of cervical spine, foot reflexology can achieve satisfactory results for patients with cervical spondylosis. It is particularly effective for spondylosis associated with the nerve roots. Foot reflexology and acupressure can alleviate the muscle and blood vessel spasms in the affected area, and thereby improve blood circulation, enhance local blood supply, and expedite the repair of the diseased tissue. In the meantime, they can also help eliminate swelling and relieve compression on the nerve roots or other tissues, and thereby alleviate or eliminate clinical symptoms.

Patients should avoid lowering their heads over a desk for extended periods of time at work, and avoid poor posture, such as lying in bed watching TV. They should also avoid holding heavy objects on their heads or with their hands. They should sleep on pillows of appropriate height, neither too high nor too low, and their pillows should not be too hard. The affected area should be kept warm.

Prescription

Do foot reflexology once daily, allowing ten sessions for a full course of treatment. At the same time, do some exercise to improve the mobility of the neck. For example, bending the neck forward and backward, stretching the neck diagonally to the left and right, and rotating the neck. Do the whole range of movements once in the morning and once in the evening for ten minutes each time.

Steps

1. Press with thumb tip the reflex zones of the kidney, adrenal gland and bladder 50 times each until a local distention and pain is felt.
2. From toe to heel, push-press the reflex zone of the ureter 50 times at a rate of 30 to 50 times per minute.
3. From the medial side to the lateral side of the foot, push-press the reflex zone of the lung and bronchus 50 times, at a rate of 30 to 50 times per minute.

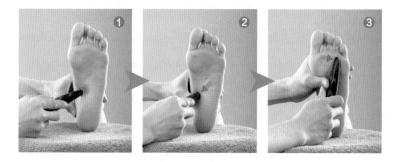

4. Press-knead the Weizhong, Kunlun, Yanglingquan, Xuanzhong, Chengshan and Zusanli acupoints 30 times each.
5. Press with thumb tip the reflex zones of the cervical spine, neck and brain (head) 100 times each.
6. Push-press towards the heel in turn the reflex zones of the cervical spine, thoracic spine, lumbar spine, sacrum, inner coccyx and outer coccyx 50 times each. Push-press one reflex zone to the next in the sequence until all the reflex zones are stimulated, and this is considered once, at a rate of 30 to 50 times per minute.

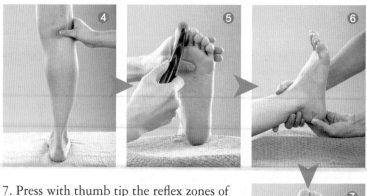

7. Press with thumb tip the reflex zones of the shoulder, trapezius, lymph nodes of the head and neck region, upper arm and parathyroid gland 50 times each, until a local distention and pain is felt.
Conclusion: Repeat Steps 1 through 3, reducing the number of stimulations by half to complete the session.

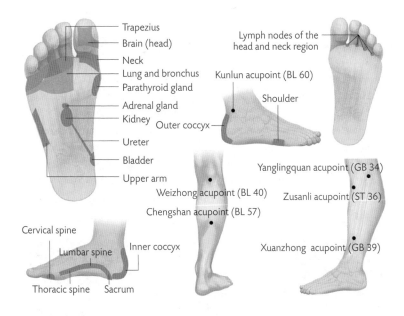

Trapezius
Brain (head)
Neck
Lung and bronchus
Parathyroid gland
Adrenal gland
Kidney
Outer coccyx
Ureter
Bladder
Upper arm

Lymph nodes of the head and neck region
Kunlun acupoint (BL 60)
Shoulder

Yanglingquan acupoint (GB 34)
Weizhong acupoint (BL 40)
Zusanli acupoint (ST 36)
Chengshan acupoint (BL 57)

Cervical spine
Lumbar spine
Inner coccyx
Thoracic spine   Sacrum

Xuanzhong acupoint (GB 39)

37. Acute Lower Back Strain and Sprains

Within 24 hours of the injury, the patient must not use a heat
compress on the injured lower back to avoid exacerbating internal
bleeding. After 24 hours, heat compresses can be used on the
affected area, once daily for 10 minutes each time. Be aware of the
water temperature to prevent burning the skin. Foot reflexology
can relax the tendons and activate the meridians, promote blood
circulation, and relieve pain. It has a good curative effect on treating
acute lower back strain and sprains. During foot reflexology
treatment, patients should sleep on a hard board bed and restrict
the movement of the lower back for three or four days.

Prescription
Do foot reflexology once or twice daily. Patients will generally see
symptoms greatly improve after a 3- or 5-day treatment. If they
continue and do 30 to 50 more sessions, the results achieved will
be greater. At the onset of severe pain, press with thumb tip the
Weizhong and Chengshan acupoints to alleviate the pain.

Steps

1. Press with thumb tip forcefully the Weizhong, Chengshan, Kunlun, Yanglingquan and Taichong acupoints 30 to 50 times. The pressure applied by the hand should generate a strong local distention and pain that is hard to bear. In the meantime, patients are required to take their own initiative to exercise their lower back by swaying it back and forth. The amplitude of swaying can increase as the patient's conditions improve.

2. Press with thumb tip the reflex zones of the kidney and bladder 50 times each until a local distention and pain is felt.

3. From toe to heel, push-press the reflex zone of the ureter 50 times at a rate of 30 to 50 times per minute.

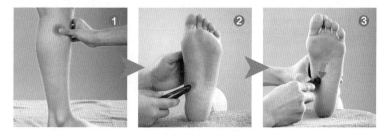

4. From the medial side to the lateral side of the foot, push-press the reflex zone of the lung and bronchus 50 times, at a rate of 30 to 50 times per minute.

5. Push-press towards the heel the reflex zones of the thoracic spine, lumbar spine, sacrum, inner coccyx and outer coccyx 100 times, at a rate of 30 to 50 times per minute.

6. Press with thumb tip the reflex zone of the parathyroid gland 50 times, until a local distention and pain is felt.

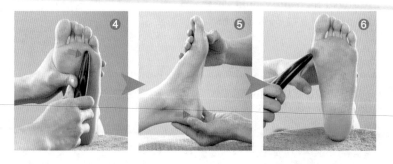

Conclusion: Repeat Steps 2 through 4, reducing the number of stimulations by half to complete the session.

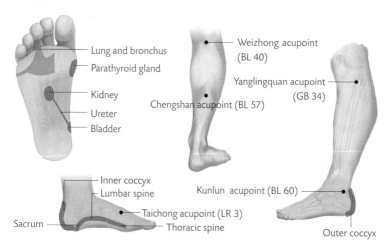

Lung and bronchus

Parathyroid gland

Kidney

Ureter

Bladder

Weizhong acupoint
(BL 40)

Yanglingquan acupoint
(GB 34)

Chengshan acupoint (BL 57)

Inner coccyx

Lumbar spine

Sacrum

Taichong acupoint (LR 3)

Thoracic spine

Kunlun acupoint (BL 60)

Outer coccyx

38. Chronic Lumbar Muscle Strain

Foot reflexology therapy is effective for the wear and tear of soft tissues in the lower back. It can nourish and tone the liver and kidneys, relax the rigidity of tendons, reinvigorate the bones, dredge the meridians to relieve pain, and boost the body's immune system, which contributes to patients' recovery.

Patients should constantly change postures at work and correct bad habits in their posture that have developed over time. It is better to sleep on a hard, wooden-board bed at night, and wear a wide waist belts for support during the day. Patients should also do exercise to increase the strength of the lumbar muscles and decrease possible wear and tear of these muscles. Commonly-used exercise for lumbar muscles include lying on the back and lifting the abdomen, and lying on the stomach lifting the head and the legs like a jumping fish. Do these exercises 5 to 10 times in the morning and in the evening.

Prescription

Do foot reflexology once every day, allowing ten sessions for a full course of treatment. After a number of courses, reduce the number of stimulations a little or by half if the symptoms have evidently been alleviated, but continue doing the treatment to enhance the result achieved and prevent recurrence of the ailment.

Steps

1. Press with thumb tip in turn the reflex zones of the kidney, liver, adrenal gland and bladder 100 times each until a local ache and distention is felt.
2. From toe to heel, push-press the reflex zone of the ureter 50 times at a rate of 30 to 50 times per minute.
3. From the medial side to the lateral side of the foot, push-press the reflex zone of the lung and bronchus 50 times, at a rate of 30 to 50 times per minute.

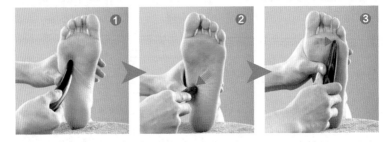

4. Press-knead the Yanglingquan, Weizhong, Xuanzhong, Kunlun, Chengshan and Yongquan acupoints, until a local ache and distention is felt.
5. Moving towards the heel, push-press the reflex zones of the lumbar spine and sacrum 100 times, at a rate of 30 to 50 times per minute.

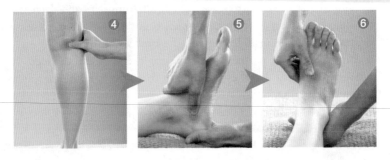

6. Press with thumb tip the reflex zones of the lymph nodes of the head and neck region, thoracic lymph node, abdominal lymph node and pelvic lymph node 50 times each, until a local ache and distention is felt.

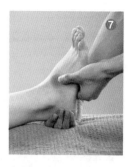

7. Press with thumb tip reflex zone of the solar plexus 20 times, until a local ache and distention is felt.

Conclusion: Repeat Steps 1 through 3, reducing the number of stimulations by half to complete the session.

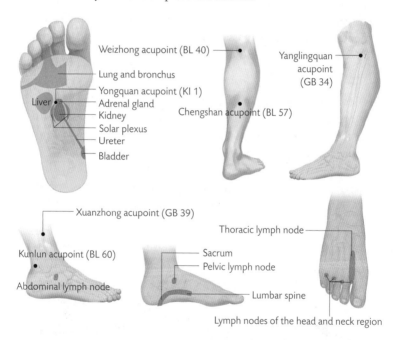

Weizhong acupoint (BL 40)

Lung and bronchus

Yanglingquan acupoint (GB 34)

Yongquan acupoint (KI 1)

Liver

Adrenal gland

Kidney

Chengshan acupoint (BL 57)

Solar plexus

Ureter

Bladder

Xuanzhong acupoint (GB 39)

Thoracic lymph node

Kunlun acupoint (BL 60)

Sacrum

Pelvic lymph node

Abdominal lymph node

Lumbar spine

Lymph nodes of the head and neck region

39. Sciatica

Foot reflexology can regulate and improve the function of the whole body and dredge and channel the meridian qi of the affected area, thus strengthening blood circulation and promoting the recovery of the function of the nerves.

Patients should keep warm and stay dry, so as to prevent an attack of wind and dampness. Increase physical exercise, such as doing lumbar muscle exercise or tai chi. Pay special attention to the kind of activities the patient engages in and the postures at work. During the onset of the disease, it is better to sleep in a hard bed and rest, which is conducive to helping relieve the symptoms, but do not rest in bed for too long, i.e., no longer than four weeks. When the symptoms are relieved, get out of bed and gradually start to do exercise.

Prescription
Do foot reflexology once daily, allowing ten sessions for a course of treatment. Most patients need three to four courses of treatment. When accompanied by massaging the affected limbs once daily for 10 to 20 minutes, the results will be even greater.

Steps
1. Press with thumb tip in turn the reflex zones of the kidney, bladder, sciatic nerve and adrenal gland 100 times until a local distention and pain is felt.
2. From toe to heel, push-press the reflex zone of the ureter 100 times at a rate of 30 to 50 times per minute.
3. From the medial side to the lateral side of the foot, push-press the reflex zone of the lung and bronchus 50 times, at a rate of 30 to 50 times per minute.

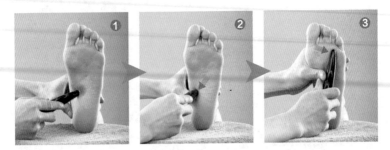

4. Press-knead the Weizhong, Yanglingquan, Chengshan and Chengjin acupoints 30 times each, while grip-pinching the Kunlun and Taixi acupoints 30 times each, until a local distention and pain is felt.

5. Moving towards the heel, push-press the reflex zones of the cervical spine, thoracic spine, lumbar spine, sacrum, inner coccyx and outer coccyx 50 times. Push-press one reflex zone to the next in the sequence until all the reflex zones are stimulated, forming one round, at a rate of 30 to 50 times per minute.
6. Press with thumb tip the reflex zones of the knee joint and the lower abdomen 30 times each, until a local distention and pain is felt.

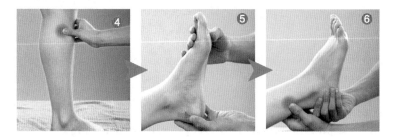

Conclusion: Repeat Steps 1 through 3 to complete the session.

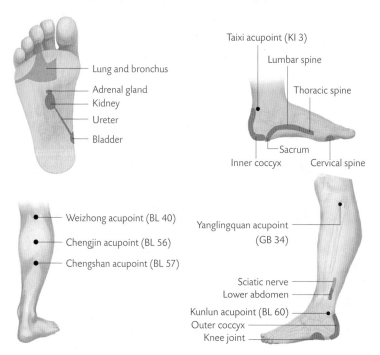

40. Rheumatoid Arthritis

Foot reflexology therapy is often used as an auxiliary method for the treatment of rheumatoid arthritis. If used long term, combined with medication and therapeutic exercise, foot reflexology can stop the aggravation of the disease. Foot reflexology can boost the human immune system, improve the blood circulation of the affected area, and eliminate local inflammation, thereby relieving the symptoms of the ailment.

Prescription
Do foot reflexology once daily, allowing one month for a course of treatment.

Steps
1. Press with thumb tip in turn the reflex zones of the pituitary gland, kidney, liver, adrenal gland, bladder and parathyroid gland 100 times each until a local distention and pain is felt.
2. From toe to heel, push-press the reflex zone of the ureter 100 times at a rate of 30 to 50 times per minute.
3. From the medial side to the lateral side of the foot, push-press the reflex zone of the lung and bronchus 50 times, at a rate of 30 to 50 times per minute.

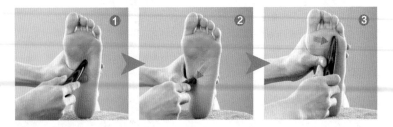

4. Press-knead the Weizhong, Zusanli, Yanglingquan, Xuanzhong, Taixi and Yongquan acupoints 50 times each, at a rate of 30 to 50 times per minute.
5. Moving towards the heel, push-press in turn the reflex zones of the cervical spine, thoracic spine, lumbar spine, sacrum, inner coccyx and outer coccyx 30 times. Push-press one reflex zone to

the next in the sequence until all the reflex zones are stimulated, forming one round, at a rate of 30 to 50 times per minute.

6. Press with thumb tip the reflex zones of the lymph nodes of the head and neck region, thoracic lymph node, abdominal lymph node and pelvic lymph node 50 times each, until a local distention and pain is felt.

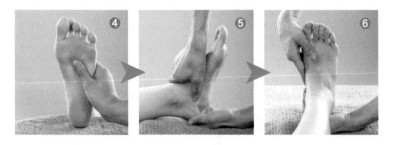

Conclusion: Repeat Steps 1 through 3 to end the session.

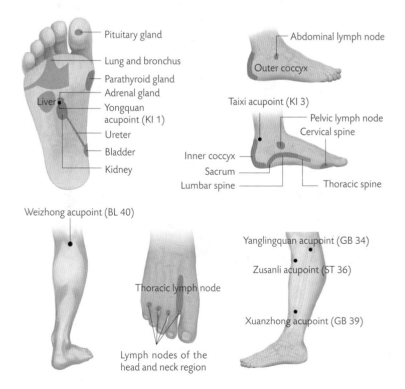

41. Irregular Menstruation

In treating irregular menstruation, foot reflexology emphasizes regulating menstruation by strengthening the flowing and spreading functions of the liver, the spleen's control over the circulation of blood, and the kidney yang's warming function to restore a normal menstrual cycle.

Prescription
Do foot reflexology once daily, allowing one month for a full course of treatment. The treatment should last for at least three months uninterrupted. Patients with dysmenorrhea should do foot reflexology twice daily a week before the menstruation starts, then revert to once daily during the menstruation.

Steps
1. Press with thumb tip in turn the reflex zones of the kidney, liver, spleen, adrenal gland and bladder 100 times each until a local distention and pain is felt.
2. From toe to heel, push-press the reflex zone of the ureter 100 times at a rate of 30 to 50 times per minute.
3. From the medial side to the lateral side of the foot, push-press the reflex zone of the lung and bronchus 100 times, at a rate of 30 to 50 times per minute.

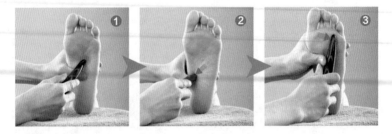

4. Press-knead the Taichong, Yongquan, Zusanli, Sanyinjiao, Yinbai and Diji acupoints 50 times each, until a local distention and pain is felt.
5. Press with thumb tip the reflex zones of the pituitary gland, heart, gonad 1 (sex gland), uterus, cervix and solar plexus

100 times each, until a local distention and pain is felt.

6. From heel to toe, push-press the reflex zone of the thyroid gland 100 times, at a rate of 30 to 50 times per minute.

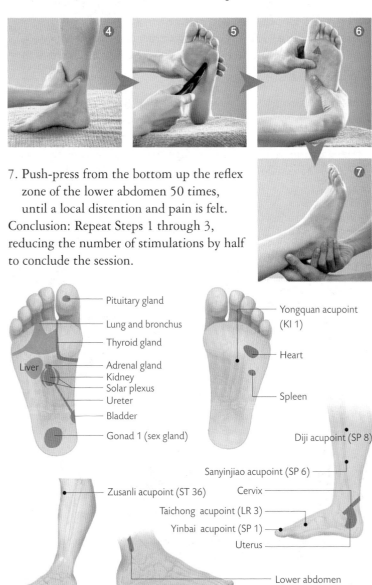

7. Push-press from the bottom up the reflex zone of the lower abdomen 50 times, until a local distention and pain is felt.

Conclusion: Repeat Steps 1 through 3, reducing the number of stimulations by half to conclude the session.

Pituitary gland
Lung and bronchus
Thyroid gland
Liver
Adrenal gland
Kidney
Solar plexus
Ureter
Bladder
Gonad 1 (sex gland)

Yongquan acupoint (KI 1)
Heart
Spleen

Diji acupoint (SP 8)
Sanyinjiao acupoint (SP 6)
Zusanli acupoint (ST 36)
Cervix
Taichong acupoint (LR 3)
Yinbai acupoint (SP 1)
Uterus
Lower abdomen

42. Dysmenorrhea

Foot reflexology is effective for primary dysmenorrhea. Patients who have developed secondary dysmenorrhea should actively treat the primary disease. At the onset of dysmenorrhea, the patient should stay in bed and rest. For more severe cases, medication should be used.

Prescription
Do foot reflexology once daily, allowing 30 sessions for a full course of treatment. Continue the treatment for two or three courses. A week before menstruation starts, the frequency of foot reflexology should be increased to once in the morning and once in the evening.

Steps
1. Press with thumb tip the reflex zones of the brain (head), pituitary gland, adrenal gland, kidney, bladder, liver and spleen 80 times each.
2. From toe to heel, push-press the reflex zone of the ureter 50 times.
3. Press-knead clockwise the reflex zone of the solar plexus for three minutes.
4. Press with thumb tip the reflex zones of the gonad 1 (sex gland), gonad 2 (sex gland), uterus, and cervix 60 times each.

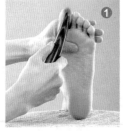

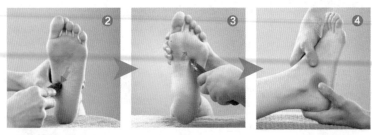

5. Press with thumb tip the reflex zones of the abdominal lymph node and pelvic lymph node 50 times.
6. On the sole of the foot moving toward the heel, push-press the reflex zone of the vagina 100 times.

7. From toe to heel, push-press the reflex zones of the thoracic spine, lumbar spine and sacrum 50 times each.

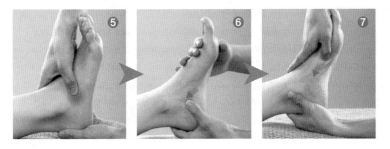

Conclusion: Repeat Steps 2 through 4, decreasing the number of stimulations by half to complete the session.

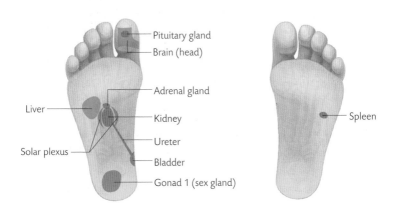

Pituitary gland
Brain (head)

Adrenal gland

Liver

Kidney

Solar plexus

Ureter

Bladder

Gonad 1 (sex gland)

Spleen

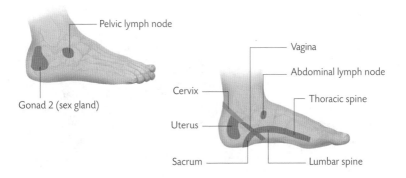

Pelvic lymph node

Gonad 2 (sex gland)

Vagina

Cervix

Abdominal lymph node

Thoracic spine

Uterus

Sacrum

Lumbar spine

43. Leukorrhea

Foot reflexology treatment of this disease is focused on clearing heat and eliminating inflammation, soothing the liver and regulating qi, and toning the kidneys and strengthening the spleen, thereby enhancing the body's resistance to diseases. Leukorrhea is caused by inflammation of the reproductive system, so anti-inflammatory and antibacterial drugs should be used. Patients should pay attention to personal hygiene during menstruation and keep the vulva clean. It is advised that patients wear clothes appropriate for the weather, maintain a regular life, and keep to an appropriate diet.

Prescription

Do foot reflexology once every day, allowing ten sessions for a full course of treatment. Continue the treatment for two courses. When symptoms have improved, gradually reduce the number of stimulations by a half. When the symptoms have disappeared, do one or two more courses of treatment to maximize the results and prevent recurrence of the ailment.

Steps

1. Press with thumb tip in turn the reflex zones of the kidney, adrenal gland and bladder 100 times each until a local pain and distention is felt.
2. From toe to heel, push-press the reflex zone of the ureter 100 times at a rate of 30 to 50 times per minute.
3. From the medial side to the lateral side of the foot, push-press the reflex zone of the lung and bronchus 50 times, at a rate of 30 to 50 times per minute.

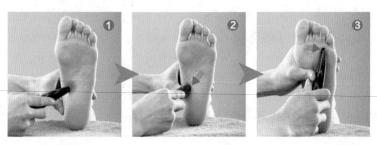

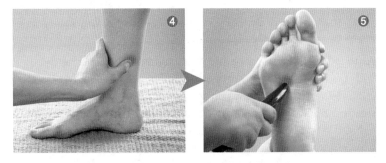

4. Press-knead the Yongquan, Taixi, Taichong, Sanyinjiao, Zusanli, Gongsun and Zulinqi acupoints 30 times each, until a local pain and distention is felt.

5. Press with thumb tip the reflex zones of the liver, spleen, uterus, cervix, vagina, solar plexus, abdominal lymph node and pelvic lymph node 50 times, until a local pain and distention is felt.

Conclusion: Repeat Steps 1 through 3, reducing the number of stimulations by half to complete the session.

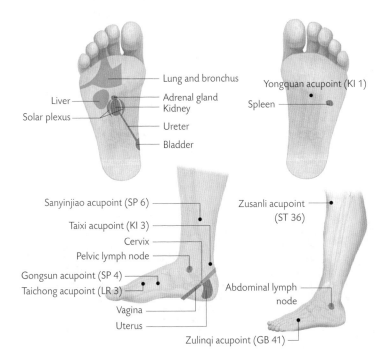

44. Pelvic Inflammatory Disease

Acute pelvic inflammatory disease should be treated primarily with medication such as antibiotics, but with chronic pelvic inflammatory disease, foot reflexology can shorten the course of treatment and bring about improved results. The patients can take reduced dosage of medication and experience fewer side effects. Foot reflexology can improve the blood circulation in the pelvic area, regulate the endocrine function, and eliminate toxins in the body, which clears away heat and detoxicates, dispels dampness, and eliminates inflammation.

Prescription

Do foot reflexology once daily, allowing ten sessions for a full course of treatment. Treatment for chronic pelvic inflammation should last at least 3 to 5 courses of treatment before improvements are felt. This chronic disease is usually hard to cure so patients should be prepared for long-term treatment and persevere in it until there is a full recovery.

Steps

1. Press with thumb tip in turn the reflex zones of the kidney, adrenal gland and bladder 100 times each until a local distention and pain is felt.
2. From toe to heel, push-press the reflex zone of the ureter 100 times at a rate of 30 to 50 times per minute.
3. From the medial side to the lateral side of the foot, push-press the reflex zone of the lung and bronchus 50 times, at a rate of

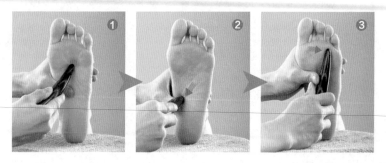

30 to 50 times per minute.

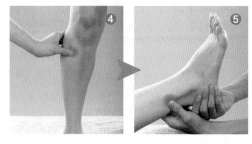

4. Press-knead the Xingjian, Zhongfeng, Taichong, Yinlingquan, Diji, Sanyinjiao, Zhongdu, Taixi and Zusanli acupoints 30 times each, until a local distention and pain is felt.

5. Press with thumb tip the reflex zones of the lymph nodes of the head and neck region, thoracic lymph node, abdominal lymph node, pelvic lymph node, parathyroid gland, uterus, solar plexus, lower abdomen, liver, spleen and gonad 1 (sex gland) 100 times each, until a local distention and pain is felt.

Conclusion: Repeat Steps 1 through 3 to complete the session.

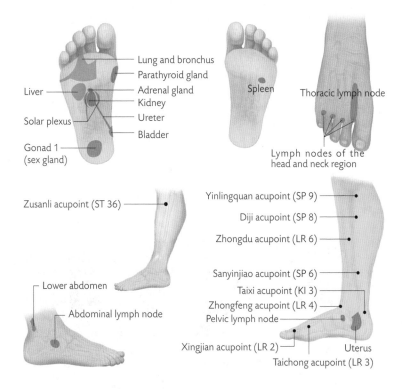

45. Hypoactive Sexual Desire Disorder

Foot reflexology therapy is effective for low sexual desire disorder. Traditional Chinese medicine holds that a low sexual desire is mainly related to the yin-deficiency of the liver and kidney. Therefore, by nourishing the liver and kidney to strengthen the function of the gonads, foot reflexology has therapeutic effects for low sexual desire.

Patients should give attention to lifestyle and diet, maintain a good mood and improve their physical fitness through exercise. During treatment, they should decrease the frequency of sexual intercourse, while their partners should learn to arouse their sexual desire and avoid acting rashly.

Prescription
Do foot reflexology once daily, allowing a month for a course of treatment. It is recommended that the patient undergo a thorough qynaecological examination to rule out the possibility of organic disease.

Steps
1. Press with thumb tip in turn the reflex zones of the kidney, adrenal gland, gonad 1 (sex gland) and bladder 100 times each until a local distention and pain is felt.
2. From toe to heel, push-press the reflex zone of the ureter 50 times at a rate of 30 to 50 times per minute.
3. From the medial side to the lateral side of the foot, push-press the reflex zone of the lung and bronchus, at a rate of 30 to 50 times per minute.

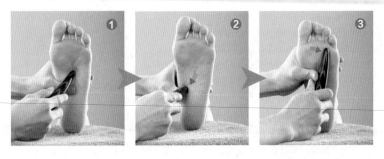

4. Push-press the Yongquan, Taixi, Zhaohai, Taichong, Sanyinjiao, Yanglingquan and Zusanli acupoints 30 times each, until a local distention and pain is felt.
5. Press with thumb tip the reflex zones of the vagina, uterus, brain (head), groin, breast, liver, heart, cervix and spleen, until a local distention and pain is felt.
6. From heel to toe, push-press the reflex zone of the thyroid gland 50 times, at a rate of 30 to 50 times per minute.

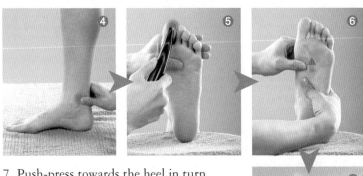

7. Push-press towards the heel in turn the reflex zones of the lumbar spine, sacrum, inner coccyx and outer coccyx 50 times each. Push-press one reflex zone to the next until all the reflex zones are stimulated, forming one round, at a rate of 30 to 50 times per minute.

Conclusion: Repeat Steps 1 through 3 to complete the session.

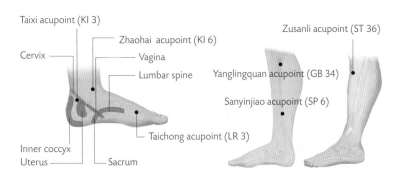

Taixi acupoint (KI 3)

Zhaohai acupoint (KI 6)

Cervix

Vagina

Lumbar spine

Zusanli acupoint (ST 36)

Yanglingquan acupoint (GB 34)

Sanyinjiao acupoint (SP 6)

Taichong acupoint (LR 3)

Inner coccyx

Uterus

Sacrum

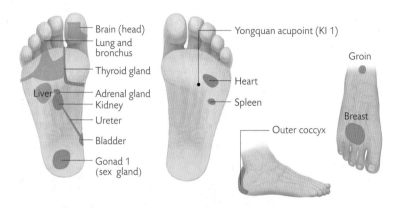

Brain (head)
Lung and bronchus
Thyroid gland
Liver
Adrenal gland
Kidney
Ureter
Bladder
Gonad 1 (sex gland)

Yongquan acupoint (KI 1)

Heart

Spleen

Outer coccyx

Groin

Breast

46. Infertility

Infertility is most closely related to the kidneys and the dysfunction of the uterus or disharmony of visceral qi and blood, which affect the functions of the uterine vessels. Foot reflexology can nourish and tone the kidneys, improve the functions of the uterus and regulate the functions of the viscera qi and blood, thereby restoring the normal functions of the uterine vessels.

In the course of the treatment, patients should eliminate mental stress and unnecessary worries, actively participate in appropriate physical exercise and balance work and rest, keep a diet with rich nutrition and a diversity of foods. They should also take the initiative to treat diseases of the reproductive organs, and limit the frequency of sexual intercourse, and improve the quality of their sexual life.

Prescription

Do foot reflexology once daily, allowing three months for a full course of treatment. The overall effect will be much greater if a full body massage is performed.

Steps

1. Press with thumb tip in turn the reflex zones of the kidney, adrenal gland, gonad 1 (sex gland) and bladder 100 times each until a local distention and pain is felt.

2. From toe to heel, push-press the reflex zone of the ureter 100 times at a rate of 30 to 50 times per minute.
3. From the medial side to the lateral side of the foot, push-press the reflex zone of the lung and bronchus 50 times, at a rate of 30 to 50 times per minute.

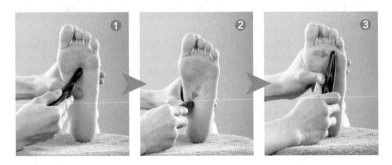

4. Press-knead 30 times each the Yongquan, Taixi, Zhaohai, Taichong, Xingjian, Yanglingquan, Zusanli, Shangjuxu, Xiajuxu and Sanyinjiao acupoints, until a local distention and pain is felt.
5. Press with thumb tip the reflex zones of the vagina, uterus, lower abdomen, groin, pituitary gland, parathyroid gland, brain (head), breast, liver, gallbladder, spleen and stomach 100 times each, until a local distention and pain is felt.
6. From heel to toe, push-press the reflex zone of the thyroid gland 50 times, at a rate of 30 to 50 times per minute.

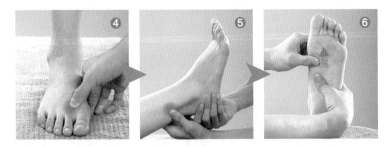

7. Push-press toward the heel the reflex zones of the cervical spine, thoracic spine, lumbar spine and sacrum in turn 30 times each, at a rate of 30 to 50 times per minute.
8. From toe to heel, push-press the reflex zone of the small intestine

50 times. From heel to toe, push-press the reflex zone of the ascending colon 50 times. From right to left, push-press the reflex zone of the transverse colon 50 times. From toe to heel,

push-press the descending colon 50 times. From the lateral side of the foot to the medial side, push-press the sigmoid colon and rectum 50 times, in sequence at a rate of 30 to 50 times per minute.

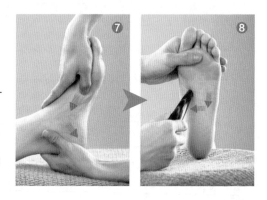

Conclusion: Repeat Steps 1 through 3, decreasing the number of stimulations by half to complete the session.

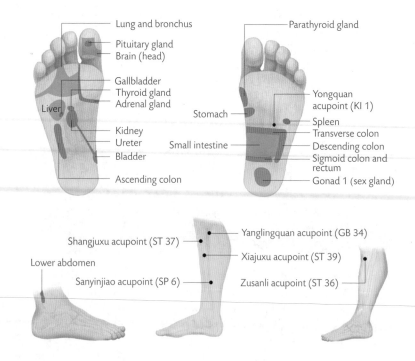

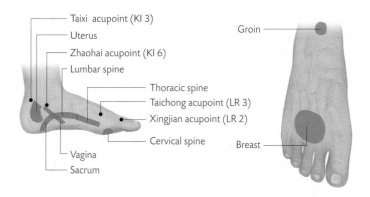

Taixi acupoint (KI 3)
Uterus
Zhaohai acupoint (KI 6)
Lumbar spine
Thoracic spine
Taichong acupoint (LR 3)
Xingjian acupoint (LR 2)
Cervical spine
Vagina
Sacrum
Groin
Breast

47. Hyperplasia of the Breast

Mainly the result of liver qi stagnation, disharmony of Chongmai (Chong meridians) and Renmai (Ren meridians), alongside qi stagnation and blood stasis, this disease can be treated with foot reflexology therapy that aims at easing the liver and relieving stagnation, regulating the Chongmai and Renmai, promoting blood circulation, and eliminating stasis, alleviating swelling, and dissipating clumps. Patients should maintain an upbeat mood, maintain a regular lifestyle, avoid spicy and pungent foods, quit smoking, and quit consuming alcohol. They should also participate in appropriate outdoor and social activities. Those who also suffer from gynecological diseases should go to the hospital for treatment.

Prescription

Practice foot reflexology once daily, or twice daily a week before menstruation. Continue for one month for a full course of treatment. The treatment is most effective if it lasts for at least three courses.

Steps

1. Press with thumb tip in turn the reflex zones of the breast, liver, kidney and bladder 100 times each until a local distention and pain is felt.

2. From toe to heel, push-press the reflex zone of the ureter 100 times at a rate of 30 to 50 times per minute.
3. From the medial side to the lateral side of the foot, push-press the reflex zone of the lung and bronchus 100 times, at a rate of 30 to 50 times per minute.

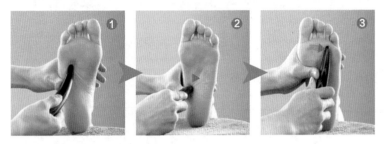

4. Press-knead the Taichong, Xingjian, Yanglingquan, Sanyinjiao, Zusanli and Yongquan acupoints 30 times each, until a local distention and pain is felt.
5. Press with thumb tip the reflex zones of the spleen, pituitary gland, adrenal gland, gonad 2 (sex gland) and thoracic lymph node 50 times, until a local distention and pain is felt.

Conclusion: Repeat Steps 1through 3, reducing the number of stimulations by half to complete the session.

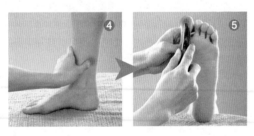

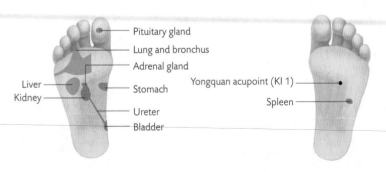

Pituitary gland
Lung and bronchus
Adrenal gland
Liver
Kidney
Stomach
Yongquan acupoint (KI 1)
Spleen
Ureter
Bladder

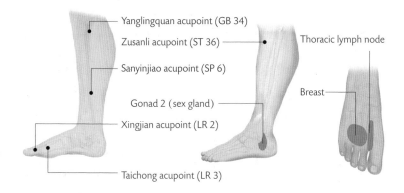

Yanglingquan acupoint (GB 34)

Zusanli acupoint (ST 36)

Thoracic lymph node

Sanyinjiao acupoint (SP 6)

Breast

Gonad 2 (sex gland)

Xingjian acupoint (LR 2)

Taichong acupoint (LR 3)

48. Acute Mastitis

Foot reflexology, having the effect of clearing lumps and reducing swelling, is most efficacious in treating early stage of acute mastitis. Those who have already developed abscesses should go to the hospital immediately. In the course of the foot reflexology treatment, the green onion steam therapy will make the treatment more effective.

For green onion steam therapy, wash 150 grams of green onion and cut into short lengths. Put the pieces in a mug and add boiling water. As the steam rises from the mug, hover the lumpy area of the breast above the mug and allow the heat to dissipate the lumps. Beware of the heat and avoid being burned. Use this method two or three times daily. Improvement of symptoms usually appear in two or three days.

Prescription
The intensity of stimulation is sufficient to generate local soreness and distention. Do foot reflexology once daily, allowing 30 sessions for a full course of treatment. Continue the treatment for two or three courses.

Steps
1. Press with thumb tip the reflex zones of the adrenal gland,

kidney, bladder, stomach and liver 100 times each.

2. From toe to heel, push-press the reflex zone of the ureter 80 times.

3. From heel to toe, push-press the reflex zone of the thyroid gland 100 times.

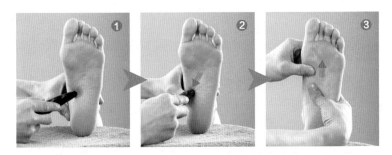

4. From the medial side to the lateral side of the foot, push-press the reflex zone of the lung and bronchus 100 times.

5. Press-knead the reflex zones of the breast and solar plexus for two minutes each.

6. Press with thumb tip the reflex zones of the lymph nodes of the head and neck region, thoracic lymph node and abdominal lymph node 150 times each.

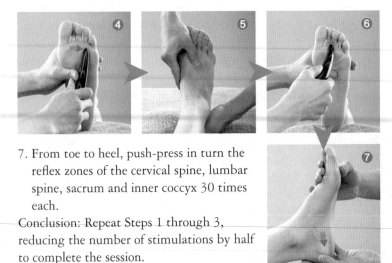

7. From toe to heel, push-press in turn the reflex zones of the cervical spine, lumbar spine, sacrum and inner coccyx 30 times each.

Conclusion: Repeat Steps 1 through 3, reducing the number of stimulations by half to complete the session.

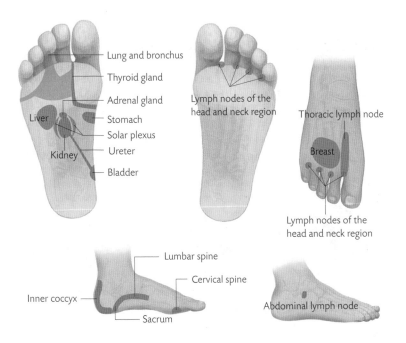

Lung and bronchus

Thyroid gland

Adrenal gland

Liver

Stomach

Solar plexus

Kidney

Ureter

Bladder

Lymph nodes of the head and neck region

Thoracic lymph node

Breast

Lymph nodes of the head and neck region

Lumbar spine

Cervical spine

Inner coccyx

Sacrum

Abdominal lymph node

49. Low Milk Supply

A new mother usually begins to secrete milk two or three days after giving birth. If the milk is secreted at an insufficient rate or is completely absent, it is called low milk supply. During the course of foot reflexology for this condition, the patient's nipples should be kept clean and the diet should be adjusted for more nutritional intake and to include high quantities of soup.

Prescription
Do foot reflexology once daily, allowing 30 times for a full course of treatment. Continue the treatment for two or three courses.

Steps
1. Press with thumb tip the reflex zones of the pituitary gland, adrenal gland, kidney, bladder, solar plexus, stomach, spleen and

liver 100 times each.

2. From toe to heel, push-press the reflex zone of the ureter
   80 times.
3. From the medial side to the lateral side of the foot, push-press
   the reflex zone of the lung and bronchus 100 times.

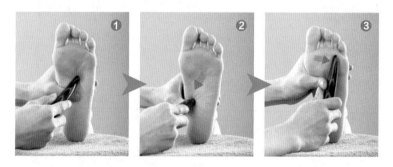

4. Press-knead the reflex zone of the breast for two minutes.
5. From toe to heel, push-press the reflex zone of the thoracic
   lymph node 60 times.
6. Press with thumb tip the reflex zone of the gonad 1 (sex gland)
   100 times.

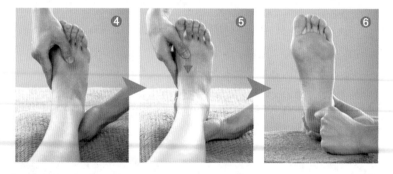

7. Press with thumb tip the reflex zones of the uterus and cervix
   100 times.
8. From toe to heel, push-press in turn the reflex zones of the
   thoracic spine, lumbar spine, sacrum, inner coccyx and outer
   coccyx 30 times each.

Conclusion: Repeat Steps 1 through 3, reducing the number of stimulations by half to complete the session.

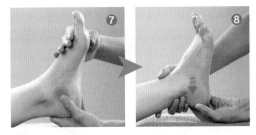

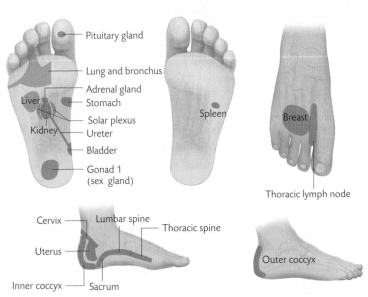

Pituitary gland

Lung and bronchus

Adrenal gland

Stomach

Liver

Solar plexus

Kidney

Ureter

Bladder

Gonad 1 (sex gland)

Spleen

Breast

Thoracic lymph node

Cervix

Lumbar spine

Thoracic spine

Uterus

Inner coccyx

Sacrum

Outer coccyx

---

50. Climacteric Syndrome

Foot reflexology therapy is effective for climacteric syndromes. It regulates the function of the endocrine system and restores the normal function of the autonomic nervous system, thereby improving systemic and local symptoms. Traditional Chinese medicine holds that this condition is primarily the result of kidney deficiency, and foot reflexology is effective for toning the kidneys.

Patients should maintain a regular lifestyle and a proper diet, and live in a comfortable environment. They should try to maintain a balanced emotional state in order to go smoothly through the menopausal period. Practicing meditation once or twice daily for an hour each time may help the treatment of climacteric syndrome, to a certain extent.

Prescription

Perform foot reflexology once daily uninterrupted until symptoms have disappeared completely. For those who have taken medication for treatment, do not stop the medication. The dosage of medication can decrease accordingly under a doctor's guidance.

Steps

1. Press with thumb tip in turn the reflex zones of the kidney, adrenal gland and bladder 100 times each until a local distention and pain is felt.
2. Push-press from toe to heel the reflex zone of the ureter 50 times at a rate of 30 to 50 times per minute.
3. Push-press from the medial side to the lateral side of the foot the reflex zone of the lung and bronchus 50 times each, at a rate of 30 to 50 times per minute.

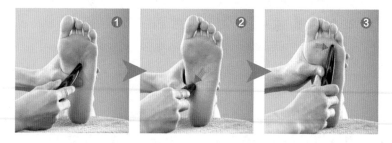

4. Press-knead the Yongquan, Taixi, Zusanli, Sanyinjiao, Taichong, Xingjian and Yanlingquan acupoints 50 times each, until a local distention and pain is felt.
5. Press with thumb tip the reflex zones of the brain (head), pituitary gland, parathyroid gland, uterus, solar plexus, heart, liver, spleen and insomnia point 100 times each, until a local distention and pain is felt.
6. Push-press from heel to toe the reflex zone of the thyroid gland 50 times, at a rate of 30 to 50 times per minute.

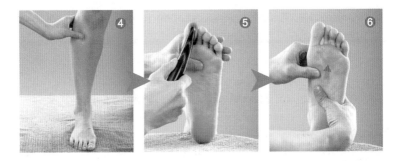

Conclusion: Repeat Steps 1 through 3 to complete the session.

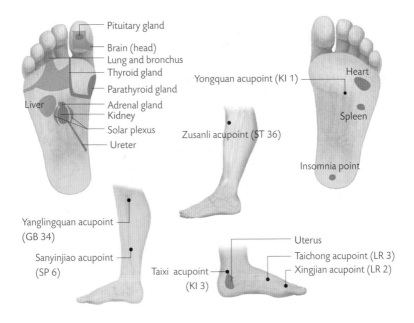

51. Nocturnal Emissions

Foot reflexology clears heat and dispels dampness, restores the harmony of the heart and kidneys, tones the kidneys and secures the essence. It can also regulate the function of the endocrine and balance the secretion of hormones. By adjusting the neuro-humoral balance, normal mental activities are maintained and sexual mechanisms are regulated, which is conducive to the treatment and recuperation of nocturnal emission.

Prescription

Practice foot reflexology once daily, allowing 10 sessions for a full course of treatment. Make sure that the treatment lasts 3 to 4 courses. When symptoms are improved, decrease the number of stimulations to once every other day and continue for one or two months to enhance the result of the treatment.

Steps

1. Press with thumb tip in turn the reflex zones of the kidney, heart and bladder 100 times each at an intensity level that generates localized distention and pain.
2. Push-press from toe to heel the reflex zone of the ureter 100 times at a rate of 30 to 50 times per minute.
3. Push-press from the medial side to the lateral side of the foot the reflex zone of the lung and bronchus 50 times each, at a rate of 30 to 50 times per minute.

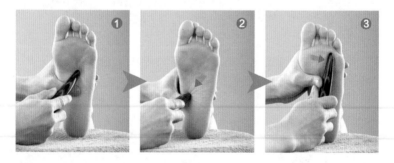

4. Press-knead the Sanyinjiao, Yongquan, Taixi, Taichong and Zusanli acupoints 50 times each, at an intensity level that generates localized distention and pain.
5. Press with thumb tip the reflex zones of the brain (head), pituitary gland, adrenal gland, gonad 1 (sex gland), prostate and penis 100 times each, at an intensity level that generates localized distention and pain.
6. From heel to toe, push-press the reflex zone of the thyroid gland 50 times, at a rate of 30 to 50 times per minute.

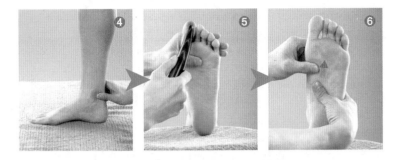

Conclusion: Repeat Steps 1 through 3, reducing the number of stimulations by half to complete the session.

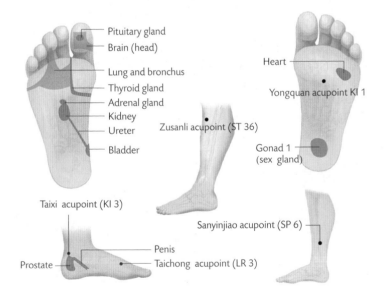

Pituitary gland
Brain (head)
Lung and bronchus
Thyroid gland
Adrenal gland
Kidney
Ureter
Bladder
Heart
Yongquan acupoint KI 1
Zusanli acupoint (ST 36)
Gonad 1 (sex gland)
Taixi acupoint (KI 3)
Sanyinjiao acupoint (SP 6)
Penis
Prostate
Taichong acupoint (LR 3)

52. Erectile Dysfunction

By toning the kidneys and strengthening the yang, foot reflexology further nourishes qi and blood, soothes the liver, promotes blood circulation, and disperses phlegm, thereby invigorating hormone secretion of the pituitary gland, adrenal gland and gonads and enhancing sexual function for therapeutic purposes.

Patients should practice a restrained sexual life and abstain from masturbation. It is important to lead a regulated life, balance work and rest, be free from stress and consume nutrient-rich foods. It is important that they refrain from indulgence in sex even after recuperation, to prevent the recurrence of erectile impotence.

Prescription

Practice foot reflexology once daily, allowing one month for a course of treatment. If it proves effective, repeat two or three more courses of treatment for improved results. The reflexologist is advised to inform the patient about the condition and help relieve the patient of any mental stress he or she may have.

Steps

1. Press with thumb tip in turn the reflex zones of the kidney, liver, adrenal gland, heart and bladder at a level of intensity that generates localized distention and pain.
2. Push-press from toe to heel the reflex zone of the ureter 100 times at a rate of 30 to 50 times per minute.
3. Push-press from the medial side to the lateral side of the foot the reflex zone of the lung and bronchus 50 times, at a rate of 30 to 50 times per minute.

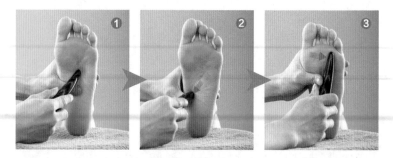

4. Press-knead the Yongquan, Taixi, Taichong, Yanglingquan, Sanyinjiao, Zusanli and Yinlingquan acupoints 30 times each, at a level of intensity that generates localized distention and pain.
5. Press with thumb tip reflex zones of the pituitary gland, gonad 1 (sex gland) and penis 100 times each, at a level of intensity that generates localized distention and pain.

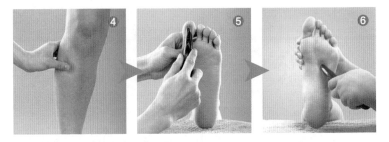

6. Press with thumb tip the reflex zones of the spleen, stomach, groin and solar plexus 50 times each, at a level of intensity that generates localized distention and pain.

7. Push-press in turn from toe to heel the reflex zones of the cervical spine, thoracic spine, lumbar spine, sacrum, inner coccyx and outer coccyx for 30 times continually, at a rate of 30 to 50 times per minute.

Conclusion: Repeat Steps 1 through 3, reducing the number of stimulations by half to conclude the session.

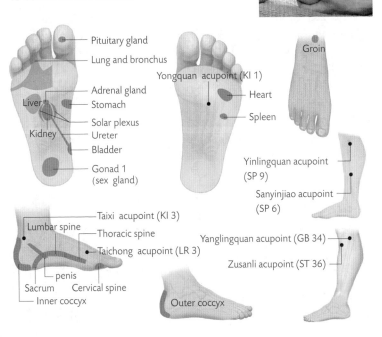

145

53. Hyperplasia of the Prostate

Foot reflexology therapy stimulates and enhances the function of the prostate and reinvigorates the function of the urinary system, thereby restoring its normal function. During foot reflexology treatment, attention should be paid to the patient's daily lifestyle. Sexual intercourses should be restrained or abstained from. Warm bath twice daily for 20 minutes each time is helpful for relieving the symptoms of prostate hyperplasia. Practicing tai chi can enhance the patients' physical fitness, but do not exercise to overexertion.

Prescription

Do foot reflexology once daily, allowing ten sessions for a full course of treatment. Improvements are usually achieved after two or three courses. Continue with foot reflexology until the symptoms have disappeared completely, then decrease the number of sessions to once every other day to maximize the results.

Steps

1. Press with thumb tip the reflex zone of the prostate 200 times, and reflex zones of the kidney, bladder, adrenal gland, urethra, and gonad 1 (sex gland) 100 times each. The level of intensity should generate localized distention and pain.
2. Push-press from toe to heel the reflex zone of the ureter 100 times at a rate of 30 to 50 times per minute.
3. Push-press from the medial side to the lateral side of the foot the reflex zone of the lung and bronchus 100 times, at a rate of 30 to 50 times per minute.

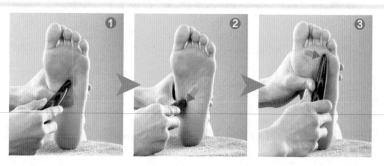

4. Press-kneed the Yonguan, Taixi, Taichong, Sanyinjiao and Yanglingquan acupoints 30 times each, with a level of intensity that generates localized distention and pain. Nip-press the Dadun acupoint 10 times.

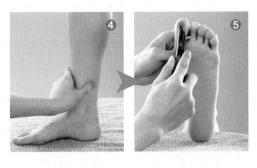

5. Press with thumb tip the reflex zones of the pituitary gland, pelvic lymph node, abdominal lymph node 50 times each, with a level of intensity that generates localized distention and pain.

Conclusion: Repeat Steps 1 through 3, reducing the number of stimulations by half to complete the treatment session.

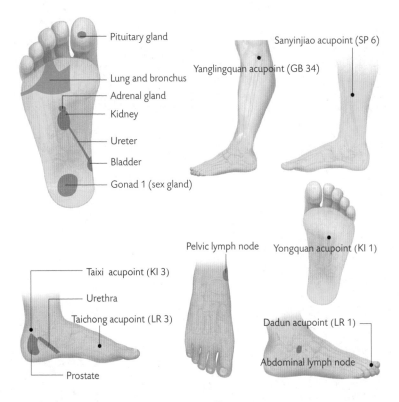

Pituitary gland

Lung and bronchus
Adrenal gland
Kidney
Ureter
Bladder
Gonad 1 (sex gland)

Sanyinjiao acupoint (SP 6)
Yanglingquan acupoint (GB 34)

Taixi acupoint (KI 3)
Urethra
Taichong acupoint (LR 3)
Prostate

Pelvic lymph node
Yongquan acupoint (KI 1)

Dadun acupoint (LR 1)
Abdominal lymph node

Chapter Four

For Health Maintenance

Today's fast-paced life leaves many people in a state of suboptimal health. This makes day-to-day health care particularly important. How do you eliminate fatigue, relieve stress, and regulate the spleen and stomach? Is it really simple to stay young through proper skin care and weight loss? Just give yourself 10 minutes a day massaging your feet, and you will do yourself a service and achieve good health.

1. Living Long and Living Well

Foot reflexology and acupressure are a process by which hand manipulation acts on the related meridians and acupoints throughout the body to regulate the vital organs and tissue and make them strong, thereby improving the body's resistance to disease. When the body is in a suboptimal state of health, it is crucial for pathogenic factors to be eliminated in a timely and effective manner so that the whole body remains in a healthy state where the "yin and yang are in harmony and health is ensured" and "positive qi is strong inside and the negative qi is unable to penetrate," thereby prolonging life.

Prescription
Do foot reflexology and acupressure once every day. At the turn of the seasons or when the weather conditions are extreme or abnormal, practice treatment once in the morning and once in the evening. Aim for a long-term practice, and you will live long and live well.

Steps
1. Press with thumb tip the reflex zones of the adrenal gland, kidney, bladder, spleen and stomach 80 times each.
2. From toe to heel, push-press the reflex zone of the ureter 80 times.
3. From the medial side to the lateral side of the foot, push-press the reflex zone of the lung and bronchus 50 times.

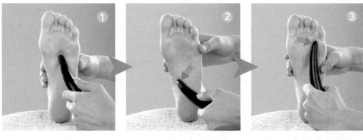

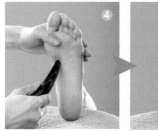
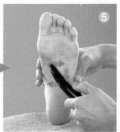

4. Press-knead the reflex zone of the solar plexus for two minutes.
5. On the left foot, from the medial to the lateral side, from toe to heel, and then from the lateral to the medial side, push-press the reflex zones of the transverse colon, descending colon, sigmoid colon and rectum 60 times each. On the right foot, from heel to toe, and from the lateral to the medial side, push-press the reflex zones of the ascending colon and transverse colon 60 times each.

Conclusion: Repeat Steps 1 through 3, reducing the number of stimulations by half to complete the session.

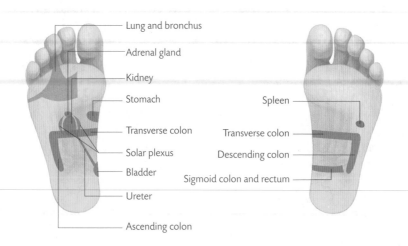

Lung and bronchus
Adrenal gland
Kidney
Stomach
Transverse colon
Solar plexus
Bladder
Ureter
Ascending colon

Spleen
Transverse colon
Descending colon
Sigmoid colon and rectum

2. Eliminating Fatigue

Maintaining health by massaging the feet can accelerate blood flow, increase blood supply, strengthen the heart's pushing, squeezing and relaxing functions, and enhance the lymphatic reflux, thereby promoting the positive metabolic balance of the body's tissue and organs. As a result, harmful metabolic waste accumulated in the body is eliminated and edema is removed, which further restores the tension and elasticity of muscle fibers, tendons, ligaments and other tissues, eliminating fatigue, removing disease pathogens, improving body functions, and reinvigorating the body.

Prescription

Do foot reflexology and acupressure once before going to bed. When you feel tired, do it once in the morning and once in the afternoon. Aim to do it long term, and you will stay reinvigorated.

Steps

1. Press with thumb tip the reflex zones of the adrenal gland, kidney, bladder, brain (head), pituitary gland, heart and liver 80 times each.
2. From toe to heel, push-press the reflex zone of the ureter 80 times.
3. From the medial to the lateral side of the foot, push-press the reflex zone of the lung and bronchus 50 times.

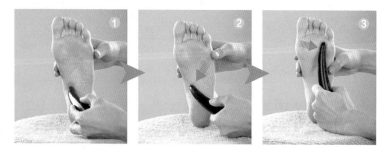

4. Press-knead the reflex zone of the solar plexus for two minutes.
5. Press with thumb tip the reflex zones of the lymph nodes of the head and neck region, thoracic lymph node, abdominal lymph node and pelvic lymph node 50 times each.
6. Press with thumb tip the reflex zone of insomnia point 50 times.

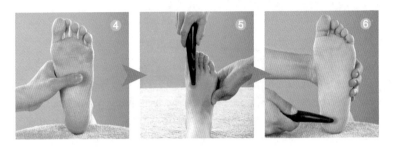

Conclusion: Repeat Steps 1 through 3, reducing the number of stimulations by half to complete the session.

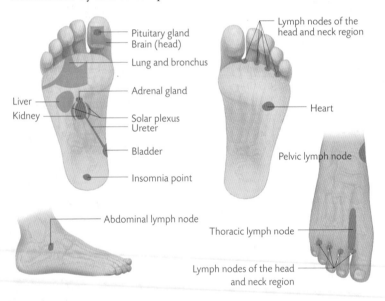

3. Toning the Brain and Invigorating the Mind

As a means of therapy and healthcare, foot reflexology can raise the temperature of local tissue and accelerate the circulation of blood, lymphatic fluid, and metabolism, thereby eliminating metabolic wastes. In addition, by stimulating the body's peripheral nerves, the cerebral cortex is activated and the sensitivity of the nervous system's functions are heightened, thereby toning the brain and invigorating the mind.

Prescription

Practice foot reflexology once before going to bed every day. For those who work with or overwork their brain, therapy should be done daily, once in the morning and once in the evening. Aim to practice it long term, and it will help you maintain a nimble mind.

Steps

1. Press with thumb tip the reflex zones of the adrenal gland, kidney, bladder, brain (head), pituitary gland, cerebellum, eye, ear, heart and liver 80 times each.
2. From toe to heel, push-press the reflex zone of the ureter 80 times.
3. Pinch the reflex zone of the frontal sinus for two minutes.

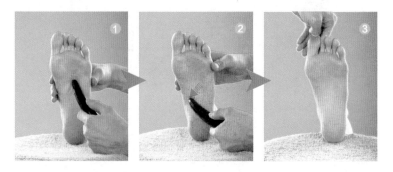

4. From the medial to the lateral side of the foot, push-press the reflex zone of the lung and bronchus 50 times each.
5. Press-knead clockwise the reflex zone of the solar plexus for two minutes.
6. From toe to heel, push-press the reflex zones of the cervical spine, thoracic spine, lumbar spine and sacrum 30 times each.

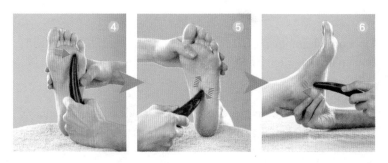

7. Press with thumb tip the reflex zone of insomnia point 50 times each.

Conclusion: Repeat Steps 1 through 3, decreasing the number of stimulations by half to complete the session.

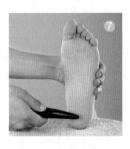

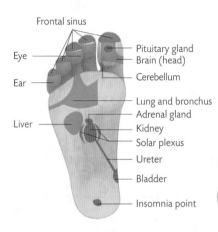

Frontal sinus

Eye

Ear

Liver

Pituitary gland
Brain (head)
Cerebellum

Lung and bronchus
Adrenal gland
Kidney
Solar plexus
Ureter
Bladder
Insomnia point

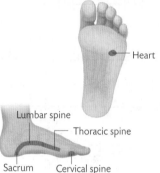

Heart

Lumbar spine
Thoracic spine
Sacrum
Cervical spine

4. Nourishing the Heart and Steadying the Nerves

Maintaining health through foot reflexology can strengthen the heart's ability to transport blood, which effectively prevents diseases such as neurasthenia, neurosis, insomnia, arteriosclerosis, and heart disease, thereby achieving the goal of nourishing the heart and calming the nerves.

Prescription
Do foot reflexology once daily. Practice it long term, and you will remain alert and refreshed.

Steps
1. Press with thumb tip the reflex zones of the adrenal gland, kidney, bladder, brain (head), pituitary gland, heart, liver and spleen 50 times.
2. From toe to heel, push-press the reflex zone of the ureter 80 times.

3. From the medial to lateral side of the foot, push-press the reflex zone of the lung and bronchus 50 times.

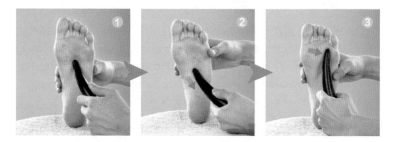

4. Press-knead the reflex zone of the solar plexus for two minutes.
5. From heel to toe, push-press the reflex zone of the thyroid gland 50 times.
6. Press with thumb tip the reflex zone of blood pressure point 50 times.

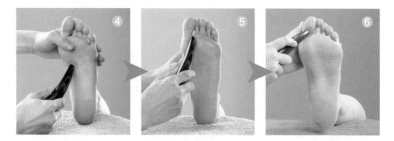

Conclusion: Repeat Steps 1 through 3, decreasing the number of stimulations by half to complete the session.

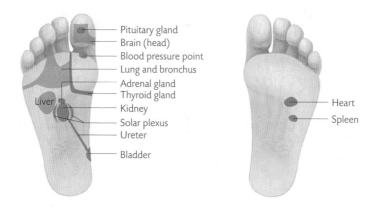

Pituitary gland
Brain (head)
Blood pressure point
Lung and bronchus
Adrenal gland
Thyroid gland
Liver
Kidney
Solar plexus
Ureter
Bladder

Heart
Spleen

5. Activating the Lungs and Relieving Tightness in the Chest

Before going to bed, doing foot reflexology therapy will activate the lung and relieve tightness in the chest, making the lungs and bronchi strong with positive energy, and thus reinforcing the body with the energy to resist invasion by external pathogens and effectively prevent such diseases like the common cold, coughs and asthma.

Prescription

Do foot reflexology once daily. When seasons change and when the weather is abnormal, treatment should be done once in the morning and once in the evening. Persevere in the practice, and you will avoid common colds.

Steps

1. Press with thumb tip the reflex zones of the adrenal gland, kidney, bladder, nose, lymph nodes of the head and neck region, and tonsil 80 times each.
2. From toe to heel, push-press the reflex zone of the ureter 80 times.
3. From heel to toe, push-press the reflex zone of the thyroid gland 50 times.

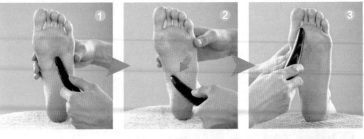

4. From the medial to lateral side of the foot, push-press the reflex zone of the lung and bronchus 80 times each.

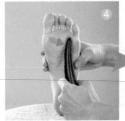
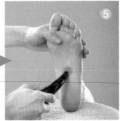

5. Press-knead the reflex zone of the solar plexus for two minutes. Conclusion: Repeat Steps 1 through 3, decreasing the number of stimulations by half to complete the treatment session.

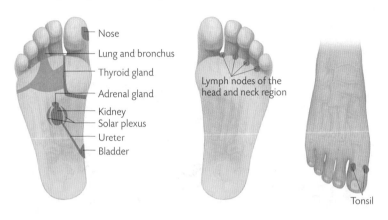

Nose
Lung and bronchus
Thyroid gland
Adrenal gland
Kidney
Solar plexus
Ureter
Bladder

Lymph nodes of the head and neck region

Tonsil

6. Regulating and Reinforcing the Spleen and Stomach

The spleen and stomach are both located in the middle burner (or energizer), and both are organs responsible for the storage, transportation and transformation of the food that enters the human body. They assume the functions of digestion, absorption, transporting nutrients and promoting the metabolic function of water and fluids. The function of the spleen and stomach can determine the functions of the other organs in the human body and the health status of a human being. Doing foot reflexology before going to bed can help regulate the spleen and stomach and effectively prevent and treat diseases related to the spleen and stomach.

Prescription
Do foot reflexology once daily. In the case of a loss of appetite or abnormal stools, it should be done once in the morning and once in the evening. Persevere in the treatment, and it will make your body strong.

Steps

1. Press with thumb tip the reflex zones of the kidney, bladder, spleen, stomach, duodenum, liver, gallbladder and pancreas 50 times each.
2. From toe to heel, push-press the reflex zone of the ureter 80 times.
3. Press-knead the reflex zones of the solar plexus and small intestine for two minutes each.

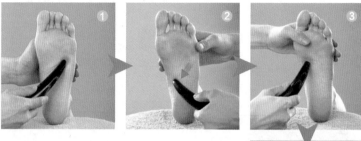

4. On the left foot, from toe to heel, push-press the reflex zones of the transverse colon, descending colon, sigmoid colon and rectum 30 times each. On the right foot, from heel to toe, push-press the reflex zones of the ascending colon and transverse colon continually 30 times.

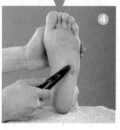

Conclusion: Repeat Steps 1 through 3, decreasing the number of stimulations by half to complete the session.

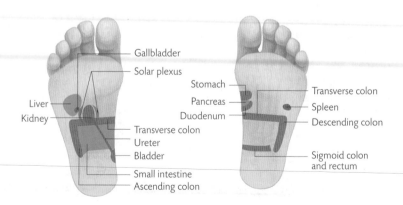

Gallbladder
Solar plexus
Stomach
Pancreas
Duodenum
Liver
Kidney
Transverse colon
Ureter
Bladder
Small intestine
Ascending colon
Transverse colon
Spleen
Descending colon
Sigmoid colon and rectum

7. Replenishing the Liver to Improve Eyesight

The liver discharges liver toxins, stores blood, and regulates qi throughout the body. It also regulates the emotions and smooths the meridians and vessels to enhance the transportation and transformation functions of the spleen and stomach. By storing blood and regulating its flow, the liver ensures that a person has sufficient blood and qi and that its circulation is unobstructed, thereby promoting the normal physiological functions of the organs and tissue. Regular practice of foot reflexology before going to bed can benefit both the liver and eyesight.

Prescription
Do foot reflexology once daily. When the eyes are overworked or during a hepatitis outbreak, do foot reflexology and acupressure once in the morning and once in the evening.

Steps
1. Press with thumb tip the reflex zones of the adrenal gland, kidney, bladder, eye, liver and gallbladder 50 times each.
2. From toe to heel, push-press the reflex zone of the ureter 50 times.
3. Press-knead the reflex zone of the solar plexus for two minutes.

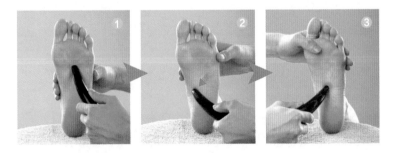

4. Push-press in turn the reflex zones of the thoracic lymph nodes, abdominal lymph node and pelvic lymph node 50 times each.
5. On the left foot, from toe to heel, push-press the reflex zones of the transverse colon, descending colon, sigmoid colon and rectum 30 times each. On the right foot, from heel to toe, push-press the

reflex zones of the
ascending colon
and transverse
colon 30 times
each.

Conclusion: Repeat
Steps 1 through 3,
decreasing the
number of stimulations by half to complete the session.

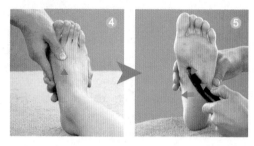

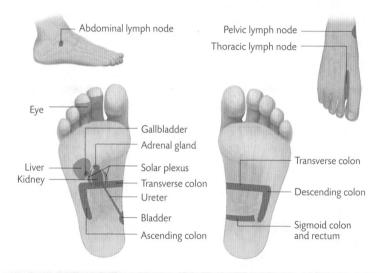

Abdominal lymph node

Pelvic lymph node
Thoracic lymph node

Eye

Gallbladder
Adrenal gland

Liver
Kidney

Solar plexus
Transverse colon
Ureter

Bladder
Ascending colon

Transverse colon

Descending colon

Sigmoid colon
and rectum

8. Toning the Kidneys and Strengthening the Lower Back

As the "inborn vitality of life," the kidneys are extremely important
organs in the human body. Traditional Chinese medicine regards
the kidneys as the driving source of life. Regular foot reflexology
therapy can tone the kidney and strengthen the lower back,
effectively preventing and treating kidney diseases of various kinds.

Prescription
Do foot reflexology once daily.

Steps

1. Press with thumb tip the reflex zones of the brain (head), pituitary gland, adrenal gland, kidney, bladder, gonad 1 (sex gland), gonad 2 (sex gland) and prostate and uterus 80 times each.
2. From toe to heel, push-press the reflex zone of the ureter 50 times.
3. From the medial to the lateral side of the foot, push-press the reflex zone of the lung and bronchus 80 times.

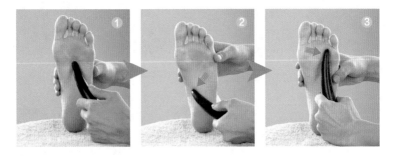

4. Press with thumb tip the reflex zones of the abdominal lymph node and pelvic lymph node 50 times each.
5. Press-knead the reflex zone of the solar plexus for two minutes.
6. On the sole of the foot, push-press toward the heel the reflex zone of the penis and vagina 50 times.

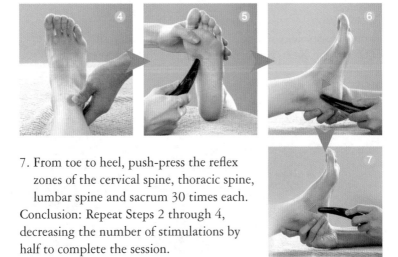

7. From toe to heel, push-press the reflex zones of the cervical spine, thoracic spine, lumbar spine and sacrum 30 times each.
Conclusion: Repeat Steps 2 through 4, decreasing the number of stimulations by half to complete the session.

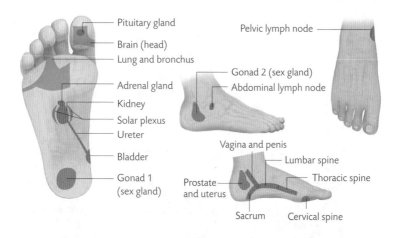

- Pituitary gland
- Brain (head)
- Lung and bronchus
- Adrenal gland
- Kidney
- Solar plexus
- Ureter
- Bladder
- Gonad 1 (sex gland)

Pelvic lymph node

Gonad 2 (sex gland)
Abdominal lymph node

Vagina and penis
Lumbar spine
Thoracic spine
Prostate and uterus
Sacrum
Cervical spine

9. Maintaining Good Physical Fitness

By stimulating the *zangfu* organs and related tissues throughout the body, foot reflexology facilitates the smooth flow of blood and regulates the distribution of muscle and fat throughout the body, thereby improving the body's shape or even reshaping it. However, to reach that goal, correction of bad lifestyle habits and an unhealthy work environment are usually imperative.

Prescription

Do foot reflexology once daily, allowing 30 sessions for a full course of treatment. Keep practicing it, and you will be forever young.

Steps

1. Press with thumb tip the reflex zones of the adrenal gland, kidney, bladder, heart, liver, stomach, spleen, uterus, cervix,

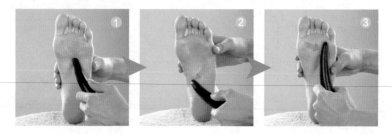

gonad 1 (sex gland) and insomnia point 100 times each.

2. From toe to heel, push-press the reflex zones of the ureter, upper arm, thigh, buttock, cervical spine, thoracic spine, lumbar spine and sacrum 80 times each.

3. From the medial to the lateral side of the foot, push-press the reflex zone of the lung and bronchus 100 times each.

4. Press-knead the reflex zones of the solar plexus and breast for two minutes.

5. On the left foot, from toe to heel, push-press the reflex zones of the transverse colon, descending colon, sigmoid colon and rectum 30 times each. On the right foot, from heel to toe, push-press the reflex zones of the ascending colon and transverse colon 30 times each.

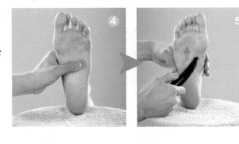

Conclusion: Repeat Steps 1 through 3, reducing the number of stimulations by half to complete the session.

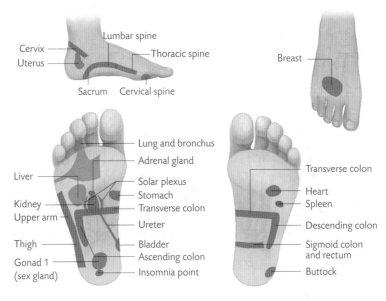

Cervix
Uterus
Lumbar spine
Thoracic spine
Sacrum   Cervical spine
Breast

Liver
Kidney
Upper arm
Thigh
Gonad 1
(sex gland)

Lung and bronchus
Adrenal gland
Solar plexus
Stomach
Transverse colon
Ureter
Bladder
Ascending colon
Insomnia point

Transverse colon
Heart
Spleen
Descending colon
Sigmoid colon
and rectum
Buttock

10. Facial Skin Care

A number of factors may affect the skin health, including high-intensity sunlight, severe environmental pollution, improper use of cosmetics, diseases and drugs. As a result, a large amount of melanin appears in the face, or the body's capacity to decompose melanin is compromised, so the face is dotted with dark spots, affecting one's appearance. But by stimulating the capillaries, foot reflexology promotes the flow of body fluid and maximizes the discharge of various pigments in the body, thus nourishing the cells and promoting the metabolic activity of the cells, leaving the skin refresh and with a beautiful glow.

Prescription

Do foot reflexology once daily, allowing 30 sessions for a course of treatment. Coutinue practicing foot reflexology and acupressure, and you will stay young.

Steps

1. Press with thumb tip the reflex zones of the adrenal gland, kidney, bladder, brain (head), frontal sinus, eye, ear, nose, neck, lymph nodes of the head and neck region, stomach and spleen 100 times each.
2. From toe to heel, push-press the reflex zone of the ureter 80 times.
3. From the medial to the lateral side of the foot, push-press the reflex zone of the lung and bronchus 50 times.

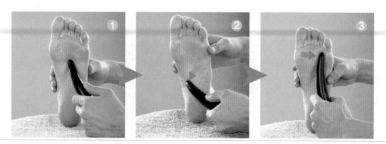

4. Press-knead clockwise the reflex zone of the solar plexus for two minutes.

5. Press with thumb tip the reflex zones of insomnia point, gonad 1 (sex gland) and gonad 2 (sex gland) 100 times each.
6. On the left foot, from toe to heel, push-press continually the neflex zones of the transverse colon, descending colon, sigmoid colon and rectum 30 times. On the right foot, from heel to toe, push-press continually the reflex zones of the ascending colon and transverse colon 30 times.

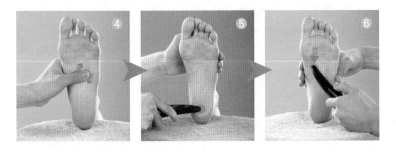

Conclusion: Repeat Steps 1 through 3, reducing the number of stimulations by half to complete the session.

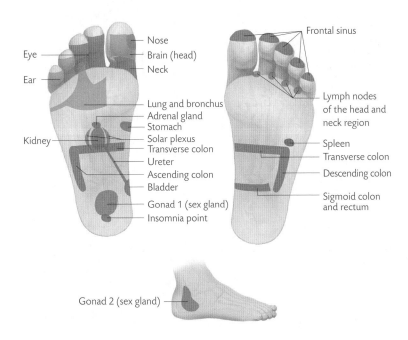

Index